DREAMING, HEALING AND IMAGINATIVE ARTS PRACTICE

In *Dreaming, Healing and Imaginative Arts Practice*, Kathleen Anne Connellan brings dream theory together with arts practice and arts psychotherapy to demonstrate how releasing the imagination can open-up processes of healing.

In this interdisciplinary and richly innovative book, Connellan focuses on nocturnal dreams, day dreams, memory and reverie, and she explores how to access, depict and use these dream images to discover personal healing. Unlike other dream journals, Connellan encourages visual recording and personal experimentation with a variety of materials and modalities, regardless of artistic ability. Each chapter is divided into a theoretical and practical half, where the theoretical section addresses the foundations of dream theory and philosophy, and the practical section offers step-by-step exercises that lead you to the creation of something restorative. Connellan covers a theme in each chapter which helps merge the unconscious with the conscious: the nature of dreaming and the constitution of the psyche, the archetype and our shadow selves, belonging, moving, pain and pleasure, and all the senses in remembering.

Dreaming, Healing and Imaginative Arts Practice is a unique blend of scholarly research, beautiful illustration and hands-on practicality that allows the reader to interpret their dreams for self-expression and self-knowledge. This work will be of great interest to those studying post-graduate psychology, social work, art and arts therapy, and an essential resource for art therapists, creative therapists, alternative psychotherapists and social workers in practice and in training.

Dr Kathleen Anne Connellan is a retired Senior Lecturer from the School of Art, Architecture and Design at the University of South Australia. She is now a creative therapist and author committed to bringing the mind, body and soul together, and she specialises in incorporating the therapeutic benefits of creativity in healing spaces.

DREAMING, HEALING AND IMAGINATIVE ARTS PRACTICE

Kathleen Anne Connellan

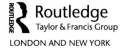

Routledge
Taylor & Francis Group

LONDON AND NEW YORK

First published 2019
by Routledge
2 Park Square, Milton Park, Abingdon, Oxon OX14 4RN

and by Routledge
52 Vanderbilt Avenue, New York, NY 10017

Routledge is an imprint of the Taylor & Francis Group, an informa business

British Library Cataloguing-in-Publication Data
A catalogue record for this book is available from the British Library

Library of Congress Cataloging-in-Publication Data
Names: Connellan, Kathleen Anne, 1959– author.
Title: Dreaming, healing and imaginative arts practice / Kathleen Anne Connellan.
Description: Milton Park, Abingdon, Oxon ; New York, NY : Routledge, 2019.
Identifiers: LCCN 2018051729 (print) | LCCN 2018055127 (ebook) |
Subjects: LCSH: Dreams—Therapeutic use. | Dream interpretation. | Psychotherapy.
Classification: LCC RC489.D74 (ebook) | LCC RC489.D74 C663 2019 (print) | DDC 616.89/14—dc23
LC record available at https://lccn.loc.gov/2018051729

ISBN: [978-1-138-71317-8] (hbk)
ISBN: [978-1-138-71319-2] (pbk)
ISBN: [978-1-315-19934-4] (ebk)

Typeset in Bembo
by Apex CoVantage, LLC

For my husband Jim and my children Mary and Terence.

CONTENTS

FIGURES

PLATES

1 Mary Connellan (2015), *Untitled Dream Version 1*, coloured pencil on card. Reproduced with permission from the artist.
2 Mary Connellan (2015), *Untitled Dream Version 2*, oil on canvas. Reproduced with permission from the artist.
3 Kathleen Connellan (2018), *The Self in Consciousness,* watercolour pencil, pen and ink on card. Author's own artwork.
4 *Tandy's States of Consciousness Exercise* (2014), collage with watercolour, coloured pencil and pen in an art journal. Reproduced in accordance with ethics protocols.
5 Kathleen Connellan (2014), *States of Consciousness*, collage with watercolour, coloured pencil. Author's own artwork.
6 Kathleen Connellan (2014), *Untitled Dream Image*, oil pastel on art journal paper. Author's own artwork.
7 Kathleen Connellan (2015), *First Dream*, watercolour on art journal paper. Author's own artwork.
8 Cumpston, Nici (2008), *Ringbarked II*, archival print on canvas, hand-coloured with pencil and watercolour. Reproduced with permission from the artist.
9 Jansons, Ivars (1966), *Near Parachilna Gorge*, oil on board. Collection of the author. Reproduced with permission from the artist's wife.
10 *County Down with the Mourne Mountains*. Photograph by the author.
11 *Joan's Mirror Dream* (2014), watercolour and coloured pencil on paper. Reproduced in accordance with ethics protocols.
12 Kathleen Connellan (2015), *Lost Child Swimming Dream*, watercolour on paper. Author's own artwork.
13 Bridgette Minuzzo (2017), *Pool*, archival inkjet print. Still from slow-motion underwater video, Sanur, Bali. From the series 'Interesting places to swim'. Reproduced with permission from the artist.

14 Marc Chagall (1887–1985), *Blue Circus (Le Cirque Bleu)*, c. 1950, oil on canvas, image: 349 × 267 mm. Presented by the artist to the Tate Gallery, London (N06136). Image supplied by the Tate London. © Marc Chagall/ ADAGP/ADAGP. Copyright Agency, 2018.

15 *Joan's Dancing Dream* (2014), watercolour pencil on paper. Reproduced in accordance with ethics protocols.

16 Jasmine Symons (2018/19), *Stalker in a Balaclava*, oil on canvas, 52 × 78 cm. Reproduced with permission from the artist.

17 Jasmine Symons (2012/13), *H-Armless (version 1)*, oil on linen, 66 × 112 cm. Reproduced with permission from the artist.

18 Jasmine Symons (2013), *H-Armless (version 2)*, oil on linen, 66 × 112 cm. Reproduced with permission from the artist.

19 Kathleen Connellan (2014), *Daisy's Collage Preparation*. Author's own photograph.

20 Kathleen Connellan (2014), *Close-up of Daisy's Collage*. Author's own photograph.

21 Residents of an aged-care home (2014), *Combined Collage*. Author's own photograph.

22 Kathleen Connellan (2013), *Beads and Buttons*, textile and mixed media on board. Author's own artwork.

23 Kathleen Connellan (2018), *Dream Catcher*, mixed media. Author's own artwork.

24 Kathleen Connellan (2018), *Baked Loaf*. Author's own photograph.

PREFACE

Memories of my childhood in a small country village where my parents ran the local inn called The Hangman's Inn are filled with all sorts of imaginative games and intriguing places of exploration. My brother and I used to sit for hours under an avocado pear tree, making highways and byways for the collection of Dinky cars we accumulated. Later I played with the fairies under a weeping willow and fed them daisy-eggs with other imaginative dainties gathered from my mother's wonder-filled garden. I dreamed up characters for my collection of dolls and designed a cosy interior for them in my wardrobe. My nights were filled with those daytime adventures, the stories read to me, and the vivid dreams of creatures and places in my nocturnal wanderings. The dark side of The Hangman's Inn, its village in Apartheid South Africa, and the long months away at boarding school fuelled a lurking unconscious that lay dormant for too long. Decades later after a reasonable career as an art teacher and design lecturer, through life circumstances I came to realise that there is a powerful part of everyone that can help make us whole, increase our creative potential and heal past wounds. This is our unconscious. So I embarked on a training course in arts therapy; I read far more than was necessary and made much more art than required, but it seemed I was suddenly on dream steroids. Upon completion of this study, and returning to the university where I worked, I realised that many of my students are starving themselves of their own dream content, they are too anxious about grades, deadlines, paying the rent and staying relatively sane. I unleashed my need to help by writing up a new course which I called 'Dream-work and imaginative arts practice' and offered it as a two-week intensive course over summer. Whilst preparing for the course I realised that there was a book in it. And here it is.

ACKNOWLEDGEMENTS

My heartfelt thanks go to colleagues and friends for providing advice at crucial times, and especially my editors at Routledge/Taylor & Francis, who believed in this book. Thank you to Juliet Newbigin, David Black, Damien Riggs and Lesley Foll for reading my proposal and supporting this book from your professional standpoints. My gratitude also goes to Peter Bishop who introduced me to James Hillman's work. Finally I am deeply grateful to Andrew Samuels for taking the time to read the manuscript and endorse it so generously.

INTRODUCTION

Dreaming, Healing and Imaginative Arts Practice is a book that serves two main purposes: healing and making art. The first aim is to dislodge parts of the self that are hidden in dreams, acquire more self-knowledge and learn creative ways to heal pain. The second is to counter creative block or inertia and discover renewed resources that fuel the imagination to develop dreams into finished artworks in whatever your creative medium might be.

As indicated in the Preface, this book emerges out of my life, my teaching and my own unconscious. As such the first person will be used frequently but it is clear when the 'I' comes from 'my' self or the many other selves whose dreams populate the pages of the book. I also often take the liberty of addressing you as the reader directly because of the personal nature of dreams and especially in the exercises for dream work. At times I use the plural 'we' and 'our' to join with readers in a shared experience.

I draw from several thinkers to assist with the theoretical sections because I wish to reach diverse groups and address many different needs amongst my readers without alienating anyone. From a scholarly point of view it may appear contradictory to use Sigmund Freud and Carl Gustav Jung alongside the post-modern views of Michel Foucault and Friedrich Nietzsche amongst others. For example, Freud's dream theory contends that all dreams are wish fulfilments and that through a reductive process of condensation dreams often deceive us. Jung on the other hand claims that through a productive process of compensation, dreams do not deceive but instead enlighten us (Samuels 1985, p. 230). Simply put, for Freud dreams are symptomatic and for Jung they are symbolic. I hope to reconcile these two oppositions and other potential conflicts through clarity of presentation and by offering different views as options. At this point I need to inform my readers that although I use Freud, I have chosen not to follow sexual interpretations but instead to emphasise opposites like Eros and Thanatos; these life and death drives combine more easily with the other scholars. The will to live and the inevitability of the death drive constitute the manifold manoeuvres of our unconscious. Therefore with these tensions and oppositions in all of consciousness, the practical sections of *Dreaming, Healing and Imaginative Arts Practice* incorporate mindful methods as a means of combining differences holistically.

The book is designed to be used as a practical resource with many exercises that may suit specific psychological, emotional, spiritual or sensory requirements. It is not a book of dream keys but rather one that encourages the reader to select tools and theories as guides to self-knowledge and self-care. Therefore as the reader, you may want to read this book as a whole or just dip into particular chapters or sections; either way all sections cross-reference other parts of the book if you feel the need to do exercises or read up on theories that are located elsewhere in the book.

I will now briefly explain the structure of the book. Each chapter is divided into a theoretical and a practical section. The theoretical section, Section A, comes first and includes conscious reflections; this is followed by the practical section, Section B, which includes exercises involving the unconscious and healing processes. Chapter 1 begins Section A with explanations and theories on what a dream is understood to be and where dream images come from. In this way the question 'What is a dream?' is central. The constitution of the psyche and the self in consciousness is key to understanding how dream imagery moves. Consequently Section A of Chapter 1 devotes considerable space to the unconscious and includes diagrammatic explanations. Section B of Chapter 1 provides clear explanations on how to keep a dream journal that consists of quick drawings or diagrams, but not text. Writing dreams is discouraged because it engages cognition and the richness of the images are lost. Chapter 2, Section A, poses the question 'Who am I and why?' to Freud, Jung, Nietzsche and Foucault. Section B of Chapter 2 addresses archetypes and shadow selves through an example of a dream and exercises that help identify and balance different aspects of ourselves. These include mask work, mandalas and a choreographed ritual. Chapter 3 focuses upon belonging and the dream place. In Section A, indigenous places and metaphorical spaces are discussed with the help of artwork as well as the poetic writing of Gaston Bachelard and Yi-Fu Tuan. The concept of temenos is crucial to Chapter 3; this is a calm and spiritual place that is separate from the intrusions of everyday concerns, and where you can be at home in yourself. Section B of Chapter 3 includes exercises on your dreams and guided meditation to assist with locating your temenos. Designing your own temenos is an important part of Section B. Chapter 4 concerns movement in dreams. Section A first deals with combined movement that is both free and frozen. This is followed with separate attention to swimming, flying, running and climbing dreams. Dream examples and artworks support the discussions of the different movement dreams in Section A. Anthony Vidler and James Hillman are included with Nietzsche, Freud and Jung in discussions of escaping and returning. Section B begins with a dancing dream as an example for analysing a movement dream of your own.

This is followed with an exercise on the 'epic life journey' and the 'flight of the soul' as a means of facing life's challenges, and returning to safety with renewed strength and peace. Chapter 5 deals with the object of crisis through theories of sublimation and the fetish. Section A engages with the topic through Freud, Jacques Lacan and Jung to identify pain and loss. Artwork is used to illustrate the ambiguous nature of absence and presence. The imagined object becomes central to transference from the absent to the present. This transference is developed in the exercises in Section B of Chapter 5 where the work of the Surrealists is central. Chapter 6 returns us more fully to our sensory bodies and emphasises the senses of taste, smell, touch and sound rather than the conventionally privileged sense of sight. Similar to the movement dreams in Chapter 4, the senses are dealt with separately in Section A of Chapter 6, beginning with the olfactory, followed by touch, sound and finally sight which is inverted to an inner seeing. In Section A, the writing of Marcel Proust joins with Maurice Merleau-Ponty and Hal Foster amongst others to challenge the mind – body split. A case study from a dementia unit is used to illustrate sensory memory retrieval. The exercises in Section B are particularly indulgent as a culmination to the book. These include harvesting and collaging your senses, meditating with sound, gardening, cooking and mindful eating.

The dream illustrations and examples, in both image and text, are generously provided with consent from my students and approved for use in this book by my university's ethics committee. I also include a number of my own images but wherever additional images are included, copyright and consents have been granted. Art materials required for each practical exercise are included for each chapter; however, it is recommended that a basic kit of art materials is purchased for your own creative flexibility. We sleep for about a third of our lives; therefore I venture to say that at least a third of our being is an untapped personal resource which with the help of this book you might be able to use for personal growth.

Reference

Samuels, A. (1985), *Jung and the Post-Jungians*, Routledge & Kegan Paul, New York.

1

WHAT IS A DREAM?

Keeping a dream journal

Introduction

This chapter is in two sections. The first is theoretical and includes a brief illustrated dream narrative, followed by explanations of the dream through the psyche and self.[1] The second is practical, and includes exercises in states of consciousness and instructions for keeping a dream image journal. Section A addresses the nature, content and possible causes of dreams. In order to do this the constitution of the psyche and self in consciousness is illustrated both diagrammatically and theoretically using Sigmund Freud, Carl Gustav Jung, Jacques Lacan and Maurice Merleau-Ponty. Section B puts theory into practice by privileging the unconscious and providing methods to access imagery from both reverie and nocturnal dreaming. A holistic merging of the body and psyche is encouraged. This is done through mindful preparation so that images from the preconscious can be retrieved through visualisation.

Section A: Theory: conscious reflections on dreaming and being

A dream narrative

> I was running uphill in 40C heat, it was a busy sidewalk in the centre of the city and I saw a man dressed completely in black sitting on his haunches, his head bent. As I drew closer I saw the thin grey ponytail tied tightly back from his face. I knew this man. I stopped to talk. He spoke earnestly about another man who was coming from afar to work with him on a project. Out of time that other man appeared, also in black but slightly more charcoal and of a bigger build. I noticed the power differentials, who will be in charge I thought? And smiling at both of them kindly, I continued my run in the heat but now the lights of the city had dimmed and I ran across the beaming headlamps of vehicles. I turned and looked back.

All of sudden my dream took me to another meeting with the man in black, I was no longer running. He explained how difficult it was to work in a team and how sad but also happy he had felt when he saw me running off into the dark with the city lights around me.

Figure 1.1 is a pencil drawing I did as soon as I opened my eyes after the above nocturnal dream. Figure 1.2 is a more developed version, a few hours after processing. This dream is now used as an example for the central question of this chapter: What constitutes a dream and what sets it apart from alert cognition? I make use of both Jung and Freud, pointing out their differences when appropriate. First, I propose the Jungian position that a dream cannot be understood without its antecedents in the conscious. In this way the dream is a 'psychic product' (Jung 2002, p. 27). To capture this product of my unconscious I sketched a line drawing into a dream journal at my bedside before waking fully. To arrive at some understanding of the personal significance of one's dream it is important to remain open to the relationships between form, movement and dialogue in the dream image captured. Second, remember that there are no sets of dream keys that are universal to dreams, and their meaning is never fixed. Jung notes, 'theoretically the whole of a person's previous life-experience might be found in every dream' (2002, p. 28). Additionally Freud notes that 'in every dream we may find reference to the experiences of the *preceding day*' (1997, p. 71). This book cautions against singular and general interpretations of dreams and instead encourages the reader to discover the psychic inferences individually through practice and exploration. For example, taking myself as the dreamer in this first example there

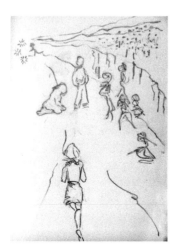

FIGURE 1.1 Kathleen Connellan (2016), *Running Dream Version 1*, graphite pencil on paper.

Author's own artwork.

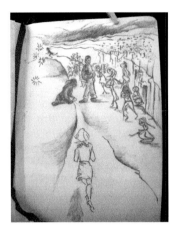

FIGURE 1.2 Kathleen Connellan (2016), *Running Dream Version 2,* graphite pencil on paper.

Author's own artwork.

are some things that immediately seem obvious. These include: I like running to keep fit and to maintain mental buoyancy; we often have heat waves in South Australia where I live; there are increasing pressures in the workplace; the scene of the dream is a busy city boulevard and one that I walk down from the train station to work, and it is also a place where displaced people beg and where others gather at bus stops, the convenience store, or just to have a smoke on the sidewalk. In this dream image, my friend with the ponytail is in an abject position, similar to the beggars; there are many other figures present but the standing man assumes an authority. 'I' am running to and from the scene. The antecedents of running in the city return to me; I stopped running in busy streets years ago after I fell in front of a car on an evening run, and I still recall the rows of headlights beaming down on me as I lay on the road. As such the involvement of my self in the dream dialogue is visually represented but there are other voices that scream silently out of the image. For me, these might refer to escape (shown in the image as running away), non-confrontation (not dealing with the difficulties of teamwork) and empathy (staying to listen); but it is worth considering how typical this type of dream might be for others. For example, could it represent shared human anxieties about leaving or staying, as part of a collective unconscious? The collective unconscious is a Jungian concept explored more in Chapter 2.

The remainder of this chapter, which lays the foundation for the following chapters, continues to address the question 'what is a dream?'

The psyche and the self

The cognitive (consciously thinking) psyche might answer that a dream is separate from reality – thereby assuming that reality is more concrete and what is outside of reality's boundaries is ephemeral. Reality is a layered concept in itself, one that is different for every human being, although there are some shared realities otherwise we would not be able to live together in this world. But beneath, above and within the multiple realities of existence lies the dream and dreaming.

Dreaming can be explained as thought set free from consciousness, unbounded and alive. For this reason dreams can be both frightening, disturbing and exhilarating. Well-known images of troubled dreams are Francisco Goya's *Los Caprichos* series; they include 82 etchings reinforced with aquatint, which he executed after a severe illness had left him completely deaf and they marked an emotional shift in his work. The nightmarish scenes contain macabre satires of social and religious abuse at the time in Spain (Osborne 1970, p. 497) as seen in Figure 1.3, where, when reason has been lost, monsters have free rein.

Plate 1 in the colour-plate section at the back of the book also represents a dream state, but perhaps one that is more exhilarating than the dark Goya image; it is symbolic of new energy and beginnings. The colour is crucial here, with red forging through the darkness of indigo but backlit with shards of yellow. Waves of colour symbolically rush forth with frightening energy that burst out of the picture plane as if this is a fragment of much more. The image was initially sketched very quickly in one session, thereby capturing the immediacy of the dream content. Later the work (Plate 2 in the colour-plate section) was solidified with thicker layers of colour which contain the emotion with intensified power.

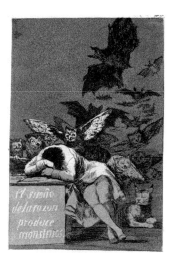

FIGURE 1.3   Goya y Lucientes, Francisco de (1746–1828). *The Sleep of Reason Produces Monsters* (*El sueño de la razon produce monstruos*). 1799. Etching, aquatint, drypoint, and burin, image: 8 7/16 × 5 7/8 in. (21.5 × 15 cm). Gift of M. Knoedler & Co., 1918 (18.64(43)). Image reference: ART322047.

All images were executed in a waking state but one capable of accessing the unconscious in ways discussed below and throughout this book.

Free thought requires letting go, a loosening of control from our rational cognition to tap into a nocturnal dream or its close companions: imagination, reverie or daydreaming. Dreams can occur at any time of the day or night although it is when we sink into sleep that dreams are usually most active. At this point it's useful to look at the anatomy of the brain especially in terms of emotion and memory which store and provide important material for dream images (see Figure 1.4).

The hippocampus is deep in the brain – it stores memory; the amygdala receives impulses for emotions and moods, which it then sends to the hypothalamus to be converted into commands for our body. Physiologically 'memories for emotional events have a persistence and vividness that other memories seem to lack' (Phelps 2004, p. 198). The amygdala and the hippocampus therefore have related functions but Phelps (2004) claims that the amygdala's responses to emotional stimuli correlate with the visual cortex *before* awareness. The importance of the visual image is crucial for developing artwork from those stored emotions and memories; therefore if the visual is held before the interference of rational cognition, it contains a 'purer' message from the unconscious.

Let us consider these movements of the psyche a bit more. The brain holds memories that we might not have processed but which are held in memory through stimuli that the body has sent. One can conceive of this site for memories as a place where aspects of our lives are stowed away but in dreaming they are retrieved without our conscious cognition deliberately calling them out of hiding. They escape and morph into characters, landscapes, interiors, objects, crowded scenes and isolated

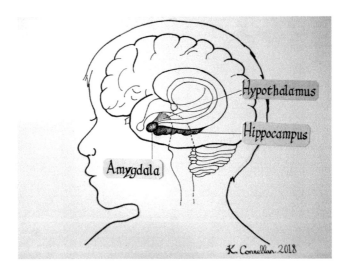

FIGURE 1.4 Kathleen Connellan (2018), *The Brain Showing Memory and Emotional Centres*, pen and ink on card.

Author's own artwork.

spaces, all with the colour, shape and sound that our unconscious gives them. However, Jung (Jung et al. 1979, pp. 26–27) says that 'the images and ideas that dreams contain cannot possibly be explained solely in terms of memory'. Dreams can express new thoughts that have never yet reached the threshold of consciousness. And for Freud, dreams are dislodged[2] memories of childhood tied to unconscious needs and fears. In this way dreams may be fulfilling secret desires. Dreams for Freud move from the unconscious to the preconscious followed by censorship, then into perception and the conscious. Movement in the Freudian psyche is crucially reliant on its constituents, which are the id, the ego and the superego (Freud 1962).

The id (the it – *das Es*) is instinctual and impulsive; it is the pleasure principle desiring gratification. The ego (the I – *das Ich*) is less primal; it is the reality principle and represents the self or the 'I' as entering into society and language. The superego (the over I – *das Über Ich*) is the sense of right and wrong, as well as the ideal self; it mediates between the ego and the id. The superego is often conflated with the conscience.

Freud is clear that the realm of the id is in the unconscious but that the ego is only partially conscious, stating that the ego is extremely influenced by the id especially in early stages of life. Freud writes, 'originally the ego includes everything but later separates' (1963, p. 5). The id, which I have shown diagrammatically in Plate 3 in the colour-plate section, is in the depths of the unconscious and has the ability to radiate farther out; for this reason I have drawn broken concentric circles around it. Freud says the 'lower portion' of the ego 'merges into' the id but that it's difficult to position the superego (1962, p. 14). Despite this, he does claim that the superego is more deeply unconscious than the ego because it deals with the urges of the id in an attempt overcome the ego. The extent that parts of the self contribute to healing through the art processing of dreams varies depending on the psychic energies involved in the dream narrative.

The id is where primary thought processes occur and this is also true of the dream; the dream is a primary processing site, where the id is active. However, primary thought processes are usually unacceptable to the adult conscious psyche and they are censored by the superego before they reveal themselves and compromise us in a disciplined society. For Freud, there are two types of content to the dream: the manifest and the latent. The manifest content is the clear imagery present upon waking. The latent content holds the deeper meaning of the dream – the forbidden thoughts and unconscious desires or fears; these images are less obvious upon waking. Dreams are generated from the impetus of the 'concurrent actions' of 'psychical forces' (Freud 1971, p. 1). Therefore, if one accepts Freud's position here, those parts of the dream that appear most insignificant provide more insight because they hold the deepest content.

The unconscious (see Plate 3) is what we are concerned with when looking into the dream and its dreaming. When the unconscious is activated dream narratives are released. The unconscious realm is larger than the conscious but this differs from person to person. I suggest that we should not try to establish an average division/threshold of the conscious and unconscious in terms of well-being because we can become unwell both by suppressing the unconscious *and* by fighting the conscious – these balances are all relative to our unique chemistries and their histories. However, for clarity of representation and, in line with the frequent 'iceberg' illustrations emanating from Freud's explanations of the unconscious, my diagram (Plate 3) positions the horizon zone of consciousness at approximately one third of the sphere. Expanded explanations of this diagram follow.

I will now elaborate on my diagram with theoretical references. First, the title of the diagram is 'The Self *in* Consciousness'; consciousness here incorporates all possible levels of consciousness and is not confined to the conscious.[3] The self and its subjectivity is at the heart of consciousness; consciousness therefore combines the mind and the senses within both a social and spiritual realm.

Several related positions of the self are illustrated in my spherical diagram which I indicate as unfixed and moving because of frequent negotiations between the id, ego and superego, as well as activity across levels and states of consciousness. Although restricted by line and language, I have chosen the circle because it is more easily conceived as a container of unfixed hierarchies. Additionally the space outside of the sphere is important for the next and ensuing chapters; that space transcends singular consciousness and time. Also, in Freud's own illustration (1962, p. 14), the self is an organic globular shape. I present my diagram of self as fluid, with the ego floating on the cusp of consciousness, thereby encompassing the preconscious, and the unconscious. The preconscious[4] is that zone between the unconscious and conscious and it shares the psychic dynamics of the unconscious. The preconscious is crucial for accessing dream imagery because as we emerge from the unconscious, to the conscious, in the half-waking state, we dwell in the preconscious which is still aware of the dream. It is probably safe to say that the preconscious is connected to the amygdala making it possible to access dream memories and bring them up to the conscious.

The concept of order in the conscious and the unconscious are entirely different. For example, when explaining the conscious, Jung cautions against mixed metaphors to avoid muddled messages (Jung et al. 1979). However, in the unconscious, Jung notes: 'Dreams have a different texture. Images that seem contradictory and ridiculous crowd in on the dreamer, the normal sense of time is lost, and commonplace things can assume a fascinating or threatening aspect' (Jung et al. 1979, p. 27). Jung goes on to say that 'It may seem strange that the unconscious psyche should order its material so differently from the seemingly disciplined pattern that we can impose on our thoughts in waking life' (Jung et al. 1979, p. 27), but he explains that this situation of disorder is not solely the work of the unconscious because disorder comes from order, and therefore also from the conscious. However, Jung emphasises that even when we *think* we are being rational, there is (unbeknown to us) a subliminal element that will take elements from the conscious, send them down to the unconscious, colour them differently and then send them back to the conscious. Post-Jungians like James Hillman (1979) say that we have to dwell in the unconscious to fathom all of consciousness, rather than look down into it from above. 'It's not outside of the dream images that we have to find meaning but deep inside, we need to go into their world' (Hillman 1979, p. 144).

Another influential theorist for understanding the unconscious is Jacques Lacan, a psychoanalyst also influenced by Freud. He is particularly important to this book because of his keen visuality. Stephen Levine (2008) notes that in France Lacan is considered *un visual*, a seeing person but crucially one who also sees the unseen or invisible. Lacan has a slightly different take on the Freudian id, ego and superego. He also has three actors: the 'real', the 'imaginary' and the 'symbolic'. I tentatively align the Lacanian real with the Freudian id, the imaginary with the ego and the symbolic with the superego. However, simply substituting the Freudian terms for the Lacanian terms loses some of Lacan's development upon the Freudian theory; nevertheless, as a point of departure for this book, there are some similarities (Lacan 2006, p. 853). For example the Lacanian 'real' occupies an existence or space prior to the language and structure of the social world or society. To use the term 'real' for this may seem confusing because in lay terms the real is the here and now of society, but for Lacan that is not the case; the real is more primal, like the id, and is as yet uninfluenced by societal demands. The Lacanian imaginary and symbolic do occupy the social world but they are often in conflict. The imaginary is the imagined and often desired other; it is a split of the Freudian ego where it recognises itself in an(other) and this other can be anything. There is an instability in the Lacanian imaginary that the symbolic tries to gain autonomy over. The symbolic takes those unstable aspects of the imaginary and fixes them into the verbal, as opposed to the visual, language of the imaginary. The thrust of Lacan's contribution to Freud is this 'symbolic chain' and order of language (Lacan 2006, p. 39). In Chapter 5 the object and its crisis will engage with some of these fundamental Lacanian concepts, but at this stage whilst we are laying some foundations for understanding the psyche and the self, it is sufficiently useful to place Lacan's idea of the self in relation to the outside and structured world of 'literate' society.

Both Freud and Lacan's approaches are more developmental than Jung's use of opposites and shadows as introduced below and elaborated upon in Chapter 2. In Plate 3, I include other related aspects, for example Jung's shadow selves and the body. The shadow selves stretch across the unconscious; these can be archetypal figures which echo with our conscious experiences in the world. What remains to be discussed from the diagram of the self in this chapter is the body. I propose that the body and mind are one, and that our senses should be allowed to permeate our consciousness. Indeed one of the key concepts for healing via dreaming is to suture any splits between the mind and body. Splits also occur in the psyche; this is called 'splitting' in psychoanalysis (Black 2011, p. 148) and is also damaging to the self.

In pursuit of healthy wholeness the contribution of embodiment, a phenomenological term, is vital to our discussion. Maurice Merleau-Ponty writes, 'My field of perception is constantly filled with the play of colours, noises and fleeting tactile sensation which I cannot relate precisely to the context of my clearly perceived world, yet which I nevertheless immediately 'place' in the world' (2002, p. xi). Merleau-Ponty says he does not confuse these sensations with day dreams but knows that he can weave his dreams into their colourful sensations (2002, p. xi). He explains that the sensations are part of 'background reality', an unlimited visual field (Merleau-Ponty 2002, p. 4). The role of consciousness *in* the body is crucial here because of the spatial dimension. According to Merleau-Ponty we are in our bodies, and 'surrounded by' our bodies – they are part of our space (2002, p. 43); the space outside of our bodies (in the world) is an expanded field of sensations that begin in our bodies.

When applying Merleau-Ponty to dreamwork, one can regard one's body as both a container and a conduit. It is a conduit because it allows sensations from the outside world to enter into its space but it also allows sensations from the pre-conscious and unconscious interior of the psyche/body to move out and around. These interior/exterior sensations are rich material for processing and developing the work in imaginary arts practice.

The body also sometimes holds memory of its own loss; for example, 'the phantom limb is a memory' (Merleau-Ponty 2002, p. 88) and the absent presence of this organic thought is where 'the relation of the "psychic" to the "physiological" becomes conceivable' (Merleau-Ponty 2002, p. 89). Additionally, Merleau-Ponty writes, 'We do not understand the absence or death of a friend until the time comes when we expect a reply from him and when we realize that we shall never again receive one' (2002, p. 93). However, in dreams, that friend might seem present because dreams are outside of time and conventional space. The material laws of distance, gravity and time do not apply in dreams.

Despite our attempts at wholeness of body and psyche, unity of body and psyche is not always possible and disunity can sometimes even be helpful. For example, creativity can be active when the psyche is in one place and the body in another.

The image of the Colosseum (Figure 1.5) is a pen and ink drawing I did very quickly standing at a side studio table, not concentrating and in my own world; that is, I was not at my easel doing 'serious' work. It was 1982, the final year of my

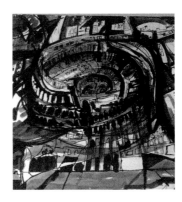

FIGURE 1.5 Kathleen Connellan (1982), *Colosseum*, Indian ink on card.

Author's own work. Photograph by Mary Connellan.

Fine Art degree. In my body, I was far from the Italian capital of Rome; instead I was in a small university town. Many years later, in 2016, I visited Rome for the first time. That is, my body went there too. In 1982, my psyche went to Rome alone and communicated its experience with dark shadows and spidery lines. Actually going to Rome helped bring a number of dreams to fruition for me, but when I physically visited the Colosseum, my pen and ink image executed so many years before seemed to have captured far more than the conscious eye could. Standing in the Colosseum I could not perceive the depth or the chaos that I had conceptualised in my image. However, what I did gain with my body being there was the smell and texture of Ancient Roman masonry and the proximity of the Forum alongside. I gained an everyday context which differed from the deep dark vortex of my preconscious drawing. I did not know at the time that Freud likened the architectural levels of contemporary Rome descending in often visible layers of historical time to our own layers of consciousness:

> Now let us, by a flight of imagination suppose that Rome is not a human habitation but a psychical entity with a similarly long and copious past – an entity, that is to say, in which nothing that has come into existence will have passed away and all the earlier phases of development continue to exist alongside the latest one.
>
> *(Freud 1963, p. 7)*

With this time warp in Rome, Freud shows us how temporality collapses in the unconscious. The meanderings of the psyche all come under the broad category of dreaming. As mentioned earlier, dreams do not only take place during sleep. All of us can think of times when we have not been present in the moment but have let our mind's eye wander elsewhere to the extent that we do not see or hear what is around us even though we remain outwardly attentive. To this end, Gaston Bachelard writes poetically of the immense value of reverie, of escaping to a place of solitude so that art and poetry can blossom. This place of solitude need not be barren says Bachelard; all it needs is a 'pretext' (2004, p. 14). This could be something as simple as a word or a sound and in a moment we transport ourselves to a place of reverie, a place of peace and of solitude (even if we are in a crowded room).[5] This is a healing practice because, according to Bachelard, daytime reverie when one is not dreaming in sleep is gentle, whereas 'the nocturnal dream is always a hostility. . . . [It] remains overloaded with the badly lived passions of daytime life. . . . It is strange. It isn't really *our* solitude' (2004, p. 14). When one is in daytime reverie even a sad memory takes on the 'peace of melancholy' (Bachelard 2004, p. 14). And so in daydreams we have more control than in nocturnal dreams where we have none; the daydream sits closer to the conscious than the unconscious. It hovers in a layer of the preconscious that can be led to places of peace if we guide the thought images carefully. 'Cosmic reveries separate us from project reveries. They situate us in a world and not in society. The cosmic reverie possesses a sort of stability or tranquillity. It helps us escape time. It is a *state*' (Bachelard 2004, p. 14).

What Bachelard is saying above is that imaginings that are not located in any particular project or work related enterprise are cosmic; they are freer and more in touch with the universe than directed imaginings. They also loosen themselves from negativity and threats more easily and bring contentment which is drawn from the soul and spirit. It is these imaginings that can be developed into artworks. Bachelard also says that these imaginings become part of the poetic/artistic state and supply us with 'the documents for a phenomenology of the soul . . . the soul does not live on the edge of time. It finds its rest in the universe imagined by reverie' (Bachelard 2004, 15).

The element of time is paramount to reverie, because even a few minutes of reverie can provide a wealth of imagery and ideas that might seem to have taken ages to formulate. Time and space become eternity and infinity in a moment; the soul and its imaginings fly in and out of our cosmos. But we cannot do this without the help of our bodies, no matter how much it might feel that we've left them behind. This is how I translate Bachelard's 'phenomenology of the soul' (1994, p. xxii). I now move to the second section of this chapter on dreams and dreaming in which I hope to bring psyche, body and soul together.

Section B: Practical: the unconscious and healing practices

Exercises

States of consciousness

The aim of this exercise is to show you the breadth of your spectrum of consciousness and assist in linking your dominant states of consciousness meaningfully. Many thoughts may be hovering in these states and they can be both positive and negative, therefore representing the life and death drives in our life.[6]

Follow the steps below to ascertain your states of consciousness and their proportion to each other. This exercise can take between 30 and 45 minutes.

Materials: a few pieces of unlined paper, a pair of scissors and a set of coloured pencils ready to use.

a   Preparation:

    1   Find a quiet comfortable place where you can sit at a table. Cut the paper into about four to six sizes, from about 10 cm square to 3 cm square. You may have some that are about the same size.

b   Mindful centring:

    2   Sit comfortably with your feet on the ground. Close your eyes or soften your focus to a haze.

    3   Become aware of your breathing, be conscious of your life giving breath as you breathe in newness and freshness and slowly breathe out *all* the stale air and energy.

4 Try to use your nose because purer air is filtered through the nasal airway. Once you have a rhythm of breathing in good clean energy and breathing out the tired used-up energy, thoughts will settle or fade and a new freshness unites the body.

5 As you feel yourself relax, notice what settles and what fades in your mind's eye. There may be colours, lines, forms – it doesn't matter.

6 Now slowly open your eyes, maintaining your relaxed state.

c   Activity:

7 Choose the largest piece of paper first; without hesitating take one or more coloured pencils to mark or colour out the patterns, forms, dots, lines, blocks, circles, merging colours, etcetera that you 'saw' in the strongest image within your psyche at this time.

8 Fill as many squares as you need to, aligning sizes of squares with strong image experiences on larger squares and weaker experiences on smaller squares.

9 Each completed square will represent 'different' states of consciousness that exist in your psyche at this specific time.

d   Reflection:

10 Arrange the completed pieces of paper in front of you, then sit with them quietly for a while.

11 When you are ready, consider how they relate to the way in which you manage your life, its tasks and its challenges.

12 Do some of the pieces of paper need to be cut into softer shapes? Like circles or ovals? If so do this.

13 Now arrange them in order of size.

14 What does the largest one say to you? Does it have corners or have you softened it? Did you use angular lines inside the forms, or curved lines? What colours did you use; did you fill out solid sections of colour? Did you press hard with the pencil or lightly?

15 Ask the above questions of every piece of paper.

16 Ask yourself which piece relates to what aspect of your life. Turn each paper over and label it appropriately just using one or at the most two words.

17 Now sit with them a bit more and consider whether some of these states of consciousness are taking up more space in your life than necessary or if some could be bigger. Also consider whether some of the forms and shapes used would be more effective if they were softer, curvier or straighter.

18 Finally, select one or perhaps two combined as a basis for a larger artwork. This work can be done at your leisure and in any form. It could a poem, an abstract or figurative painting or sculpture, a dance movement or a piece of music. In other words, you choose your medium. The artwork can then be something that encourages you to take more control of a situation, or, if needs be, to let go of a situation.

Plate 4 in the colour-plate section is an example from one my students 'Tandy' who pasted her states of consciousness pieces into an art journal, wrote accompanying reflections and numbered them according to the space they take up in her mind rather than using size to indicate this. One of the smaller images showing a round yellow 'sun' with the accompanying reflective text saying 'love of happiness, and the good things – complete appreciation' is almost hidden. She then developed some of the anxiety and negative self-feeling to incorporate positivity on the right-hand page.

Plate 5 in the colour-plate section shows my own states of consciousness exercise five years ago according to size. Here my dominant state was 'organisation', followed by creative endeavours with anxieties at the 'end'

Summing up states of consciousness exercise

You may be surprised at what takes up so little of your psychic space and yet it's really important for your well-being. Often we sacrifice a healthy practice because of work or other pressure. The states of consciousness pieces of paper should be put into an envelope and dated so that the next time you do it you can compare. It's useful to do this exercise every few months, perhaps four times a year. There are unique reasons for our states of consciousness. For example, our central nervous system has two parts: the sympathetic, which gets the body into action for fight or flight, and the parasympathetic, which brings the body back; in such a situation our pupils dilate and then come back to normal. So the sympathetic can be seen as the accelerator and the parasympathetic as the brake. It is possible to have a foot on both; however the sympathetic system is put into action really quickly with the parasympathetic quite slow. Therefore you might have seen evidence of flat states and alert states in relation to parts of your life, and it is important to recognise which aspects need lifting and which need calming in proportion to your life goals.

Keeping a visual dream journal: your resource for all ensuing exercises in this book

Materials: Pocket-sized unlined sketch book (your dream journal) and a sharpened pencil or an easy to use pen.

Sometimes it's difficult to recall nocturnal dreams, so I include other types of dreams to capture in the dream journal. Nonetheless, nocturnal dreams should be given priority because they come from a deeper unconscious. Even if you have 'never' remembered a night dream, if you persist with this journal your preconscious will offer you some dreams. The dream content from visualisations and daydreams/reverie emerge from your preconscious and are also immensely useful for healing in imaginative arts practice. Instructions for daydreams and visualisation require similar breathing techniques already provided in the states of consciousness exercise.

Nocturnal dreams

Preparation:

1   Ensure that the journal and pen/pencil are right beside your bed before you go to sleep.

Activity:

2   The very moment you awaken and without speaking to anyone, take the pencil/pen and *very* quickly sketch your clearest dream on one page without any thought about proportion, composition or quality of line – in fact, without thinking at all. Remember, do not worry if you 'cannot draw'. This must take no longer than 1 or, at the most, 2 minutes. Stick figures, blocks and circles are fine.
3   It is important to draw and *not to write* unless there were singular words 'as images' in the dream. Writing takes longer and there's the danger of returning to controlled cognition if the dream is written down.
4   Colours should be noted so that when the journal image is developed into an art piece, it can faithfully replicate the dominant colours.
5   If the dream is monochrome or black and white, try to remember if there were shades of grey, tonalities of white and whether there was a grainy, blurry or smooth texture.
6   Each page must be dated.
7   Make a drawing every morning if possible; with this repetitive practice your hand will take over from your 'mind' and you'll become really loose and fast at capturing the main actors in your dream spaces.
8   Keep your journal private.
9   Always acknowledge that this is your dream and drawing it is only something you can do. Also realise that it is only possible whilst the dream is still fresh and lying at the cusp of your consciousness, ready to fade but just as ready to stay alight whilst you capture its psychic content.

Visualisation

Materials: the same as for nocturnal dreams.

Preparation:

1   Find a quiet and comfortable place to sit where your feet touch the ground. Ensure you are warm enough.
2   Allow yourself 20 minutes and ensure there will be no interruptions. You might want to set a soft time alarm for yourself.
3   Read through these instructions but don't worry if you can't recall them all the first times that you do this exercise. After a few times you'll get into the habit.
4   Ensure that you have your dream journal materials beside you.

Process:

5 Close your eyes or soften your focus completely.
6 Begin to notice your breath, breathe in newness and freshness, and slowly breathe out the stale air and energy.
7 Just 'be' in your breath, in and out, in and out, slowly, and when thoughts come in or sounds occur, just notice them, don't keep them – they will come and go, it's natural.
8 Once you have a deep rhythm of breathing, be aware of your body completely relaxed in the chair; notice if there is any pain, discomfort or tension in a part or parts of your body, take your breath to those parts, breathing fresh air into the muscles or organs and let them melt with the air.
9 Know that your body is there in that chair, in the room, in that building, in that town, which sits in a country and continent surrounded by seas on a spherical globe amongst the many stars in the universe.

Visually self-guided mindfulness:

10 Slowly, now take yourself to your favourite place of peace which might be a lonely beach, beneath the shade of an ancient tree or inside a room of nurturing memories.
11 Stay there in that place of peace, noticing its calmness, the colours and shapes that make it special for you; be there and notice what occurs.
12 After a while, bid a soft farewell to the place and its inhabitants, once again becoming aware of your breath in your body.
13 Slowly open your eyes and wiggle your fingers and toes.

Activity:

14 Now reach for your journal and sketch the place you went to and any inhabitants and objects in it. Do this swiftly not thinking about proportion or realism. Label the colours and tones as appropriate but only after the sketch is complete. Avoid writing unless there were word images.
15 Date and time the dream page.
16 As you complete this exercise in your comfortable seat, take a moment to be aware of where you are now, and be kind to yourself as you mentally prepare to take on the next tasks of your day. You've just been away and may feel a little fragile, vulnerable or strangely distant from this world. You might need a little more time to gather yourself before engaging with others; just be gentle with yourself because even though you might have been to a place of peace, your psyche may have included other things which found their way into your drawing. These are all parts of your self and learning how to balance them is one of the aims of this book.

Daydreams/reveries

Materials: The same as for the nocturnal and visualisation above.

   Daydreams and reveries are unplanned; they tend to just happen if we are prone to them. Therefore if you are susceptible to frequent or unexpected reveries during the day, you'll need to keep your journal and a pencil/pen in your pocket or in a *very* easy-to-access place during your day.

1   You might be reading, looking at a scene, listening to a talk or doing something else where it is not dangerous to let your psyche wander.
2   Give yourself permission to daydream without compromising yourself or others.
3   Allow yourself 20 minutes; how you time this is a bit organic because it's usually a sound from this world that brings you back to the present.
4   As your psyche leaves the present, follow it with your body, but physically remain where you are, staying still, relaxed and comfortable.
5   Wherever you go and whatever the dialogue, notice the place and its inhabitants, the sounds and the silences, but let them all be free. Stay there for as many minutes as the reverie permits.
6   When there is a trigger (which could be a sound reminder) to return to the present, reach for your journal and sketch immediately and quickly, ensuring all the actors, the details of the place and its event are recorded in line and form, but do not be concerned about realism or proportion. Take no more than 2 minutes.
7   If words are crucial to a dream dialogue, note them, but it's far better to have the emotion captured through a large or small form, dots, circles, streaky lines, blocks, shaded areas and the distance between each.
8   Label the colours and tones.
9   Date and time the dream page.
10   Bring yourself to the present; be kind to yourself.

Summing up the dream journal exercise

Nocturnal dreams can be alarming and puzzling. Do not try to analyse them too much although it's tempting. The remainder of this book will assist you in making some sense of the actors, events and places in your dreams. Visualisations are more controlled because you take yourself to places, you can also use mindfulness apps, CDs or YouTube videos to guide you to a place of peace, but let your own psyche and body populate those places so that they are your own. With daytime reveries, there are sometimes delicious fantasies or wild journeys; whatever they are, all of these are a part of your being.

   In the process of daytime dreaming the shifting dimensions from cognition to embodiment lightens the heaviness of thought in the psyche and creates space/

breath in the head. Staying with the breath, your body might even take you into a painting you're doing, an incomplete musical composition, or a poem where words are finding their tempo in your thoughts. This is not necessarily 'project reverie' but a visualisation that can come to rest in a place where creativity can bear fruit (Bachelard 2004, p. 14).

In reverie and visualisation, you change your state of consciousness. What might have been anxious, sad, angry or generally overwhelmed now changes to one that can be calm and relaxed, thus allowing harmful thought-images to dissolve and healing thought-images to form.

Conclusion

This chapter has laid open some information on the nature of dreaming, addressing the cognitive psyche and spectrums of consciousness. Key theorists like Freud, Jung and Lacan contributed to these discussions. We've also considered the art of reverie through the writings of Bachelard and the importance of the body through the work of Merleau-Ponty. Dream narrations and images are represented to show examples of the unconscious. The constitution of the self is diagrammatically illustrated for additional insight into the workings of the psyche with our body. Finally, the practical section teaches us how to keep and use a dream journal and also how to monitor our states of consciousness.

The next chapter delves into different aspects and masks of our self; it addresses the possibility of shadow selves as a reflection of the everyday self and how acknowledging these other selves might lead to deeper understanding and healing.

Notes

1 I use the term 'psyche' rather than 'mind' because it is more inclusive of the soul. I owe this to Bruno Bettelheim (1984) who alerts readers to the serious mistranslation of Freud. Freud used the German *Psyche* and *Seele* (soul) interchangeably at times and Bettelheim emphasises that the absence of 'soul' and the use of the English word 'mind' casts Freud in an erroneous light and shows his theories to be unfairly fixed thereby losing an essential fluidity that points to the struggles of soul in the psyche and across consciousness.
2 Here again, instead of using the common term 'repressed' from English translations of Freud, I use the softer term 'dislodged' which is a more accurate translation from the German *Verdrängung* according to Bettelheim (1984: 93). Bettelheim notes that *Verdrängung* involves an 'inner urge'.
3 David Black (2011) writes informatively on current debates and positions on consciousness in psychoanalysis, science and religion.
4 The preconscious is a Freudian psychoanalytic term which I will use in this book instead of the more common lay term 'subconscious' which is often used to describe that layer of the unconscious which is near the surface of consciousness.
5 Chapter 3 'Belonging' includes more about place and space in reverie/daydreams.
6 The exercise 'states of consciousness' borrows the name from process psychology and also transpersonal psychology, but it does not delve into altered states of consciousness like the coma; for more on this aspect, Mindell (1991) and Tart (2000) are useful references.

References

Bachelard, G. (1994), *The Poetics of Space: The classic look at how we experience intimate places*, trans. M. Jolas, Beacon, Boston, MA.

Bachelard, G. (2004), *The Poetics of Reverie: Childhood, language and the cosmos*, trans. D Russell, Beacon, Boston, MA.

Bettelheim, B. (1984), *Freud and Man's Soul*, Vintage, New York.

Black, D.M. (2011), *Why Things Matter: The place of values in science, psychoanalysis and religion*, Routledge, London.

Freud, S. (1962), *The Ego and the Id*, trans. J. Riviere, rev. edn. J. Strachey, Hogarth Press and Institute of Psychoanalysis, London.

Freud, S. (1963), *Civilization and its Discontents*, trans. J. Riviere, rev. edn, J. Strachey, Hogarth Press and Institute of Psychoanalysis, London.

Freud, S. (1971), *The Interpretation of Dreams*, trans. J. Strachey, Allen & Unwin, London.

Freud, S. (1997), *The Interpretation of Dreams*, trans. A.A. Brill, Wordsworth Classics, Ware.

Hillman, J. (1979), *The Dream and the Underworld*, Harper & Row, New York.

Jung, C.G., von Franz, M.L., Henderson, J.L., Jacobi, J. and Jaffé, A. (1979), *Man and His Symbols*, Picador, New York.

Jung, C.G. (2002), *Dreams*, trans. R.F.C. Hull, Routledge, London.

Lacan, J. (2006), *Écrits*, trans. B. Fink, Norton, London.

Levine, S.Z. (2008), *Lacan Reframed: A guide for the arts student*, Tauris, London.

Merleau-Ponty, M. (2002), *Phenomenology of Perception*, trans. C. Smith, Routledge, London.

Mindell, A. (1991), *City Shadows: Psychological Interventions in Psychiatry*, Arkana, London.

Osborne, H. (ed.) (1970), *The Oxford Companion to Art*, Oxford University Press, London.

Phelps, E.A. (2004), 'Human emotion and memory: interactions of the amygdala and hippocampal complex', *Current Opinion in Neurobiology*, vol. 14, pp. 198–202.

Tart, C.T. (2000), *States of Consciousness: Body, mind & spirit*, iUniverse, Bloomington, IN.

2

WHO AM I AND WHY?

Archetypes and shadows

Introduction

The self and its shadows is the central theme of this chapter; in other words, the idea that we are not one but many. A secondary theme is the metaphysical space that these selves inhabit; as such the world and its universe is presented here as the context for a collective psyche. The individual self in that collective is therefore also shown to be a diversity of complex parts exemplified across the unconscious in the guise of archetypes. The Cambridge and Oxford dictionaries explain archetypes as 'typical' or 'original' examples of a thing or person, but in this chapter archetypes do not share that denotative similarity with stereotypes or typification generally. Instead the Jungian interpretation which takes the archetype further is a useful one for the purposes of this chapter. In this way archetypes are symbolic holders of composite characteristics. They are universal themes of the psyche, and this is a self that is part of what Jung calls the 'collective unconscious'. Additionally an archetype in the unconscious and dream world has its parallel in the conscious and is referred to as the shadow because it is a kind of unconscious echo of the conscious self. Jung argues 'If we want to interpret a dream correctly, we need a thorough knowledge of the conscious situation at that moment because the dream contains its unconscious complement' (2002, p. 36).

To address both the conscious and unconscious and gain insights into the tension between the self and its shadows, this chapter has a theoretical and a practical section.

The theoretical section includes conscious reflections of the self and the soul/psyche, passed down from Foucault, Nietzsche and Freud, providing a philosophical balance to understandings of the archetype. Additionally, archetypal psychology is generally considered different from developmental psychology; however, post-Jungian thinking suggests that they are not necessarily opposed because both delve below surfaces and move back and forth (Giegerich 1991, p. 90). In this way depth psychology adopted by post-Jungians (Hillman 1979) also underpins this chapter. Consequently the constitution of consciousness as discussed in Chapter 1 is expanded upon by further addressing the soul/psyche and questions of self-knowledge.

The practical section includes exercises involving the unconscious and healing processes through shadow work, mandala and ritual.

Section A: Theory: conscious reflections on knowing oneself

The profoundly simple question, 'who am I and why?' if posed to yourself in private demands deep consideration. In contrast you may recall occasions when you are asked to provide your name(s), gender, occupation, address, nationality, state of health, religion and perhaps even background information which gives reasons for who you are and why. At such times, you may reflect a little on the meaning of your answers but it's likely that you'll fill in the form and tick boxes without dwelling too deeply on who you are to yourself. Such procedures are more about who you are to others. In this section we'll deal with both the private and the public persona and how they might inform each other. However despite the potential enormity of this topic, my aim is to keep this discussion as simple as possible.

Classical philosophy and Michel Foucault (1926–1984[1])

Many philosophers over time have grappled with the question of 'who am I and why?' The Classical Greek philosopher Socrates (470–399 BCE) instructed that to fulfil one's role in life it is imperative to attend to the self first. Therefore the Greek Delphic oracular learning to know yourself (*gnōthi seauton*) should be closely accompanied with 'care' and 'cultivation' of the self (*epimeleia heautou*) (Foucault 2005, p. 44). Knowledge of the self is gained through regular practices which pay close attention to our everyday activities; Foucault notes that these practices bring the subject of the self into honest focus (Foucault 2005, p. 3; Foucault 2010, pp. 240, 241). However such practices cannot be casual or inter-mittent; a part of each day should always (almost like a ritual) be devoted to the care of the self.

Additionally Foucault says that this care of the self is not exclusively solitary but it is also and, importantly, 'a true social practice' (2005, p. 51). Therefore it is not only how we are to ourselves but how we are and how we interact with other human beings. To this end guidance from qualified and trusted profession-als who can provide counsel can help to establish and maintain practices that suit our needs; however, it is important to be aware of the power relations inherent in some aspects of pastoral care and to be clear sighted about all agendas. None-theless many people find solace in the gentle faith of kindness and in a promise of eternal spiritual life. Currently mindfulness practices are also being embraced and there are additional exercises in the healing practices of this book which may assist in gaining knowledge of useful care practices.

I return now to the importance of knowing oneself as a constituent of caring for the self. It is often the 'soul' that comes into focus in philosophical writings about knowing the self; 'looking into one's soul' or 'soul-searching' are turns of phrase that can be secular or spiritual. Referring to Ancient Greece, Foucault notes that the 'soul is something mobile' and that it is vulnerable:

> The soul, the breath, is something that can be disturbed and over which the outside can exercise a hold. One must avoid dispersal, of the soul, the breath, the *pneuma*. One must avoid exposing it to external danger and something or someone having a hold over it.
>
> *(2005, p. 47)*

The soul is that invisible part of our selves that is also the most precious. Linking it to the breath Foucault draws from the Stoics in Hellenistic Greece for whom the *pneuma* is the vital spirit and creative force of a person.

Friedrich Nietzsche (1844–1900) and the soul

The vulnerability and power of the soul that is sometimes hidden within the self is what Nietzsche, a philosopher greatly respected by Foucault, devoted much of his writing to. In his long poem *Thus Spoke Zarathustra*, Nietzsche writes that Zarathustra may seem asleep but he is actually conversing with his soul (1976, p. 333). In 'On the Great Longing', which is in the third part of *Zarathustra*, Nietzsche proclaims the work Zarathustra has already done on his soul and yet it remains at risk:

> O my soul, I delivered you from all nooks; I brushed dust, spiders, and twilight off you.
>   . . . O my soul, I gave you back the freedom over the created and uncreated; and who knows, as you know, the voluptuous delight of what is yet to come?
>   . . . O my soul, now there is not a soul anywhere that would be more loving and comprehending and comprehensive. Where would future and past dwell closer together than in you?
>   . . . O my soul, I understand the smile of your melancholy: now your own overrichness stretches out longing hands. . . . And verily, O my soul, who could see your smile and not be melted by tears . . .
>
> *(Nietzsche 1976, pp. 334, 335)*

Nietzsche shows that the soul is retrieved from hiding and brought into light; indeed he notes that the soul becomes 'as still as light' (1976, p. 334) but eventually the freed soul is imbued with so much that it also becomes heavy. In a typically paradoxical way Nietzsche collapses the sacred and the profane into a soul that is now overfull and weighed down.

Sigmund Freud (1886–1939), the soul and struggle

Freud, a generation younger but influenced by Nietzsche, was also deeply concerned with the workings of the human soul, despite the absence of the word *seele* in English translations (see Chapter 1, note 1). Freud advanced the knowledge of the psyche with his contributions on the id (*das Es*), the ego (*das Ich*) and the superego (*das Über Ich*) as discussed in Chapter 1, pursuing the idea of dislodged desire (*Verdrängung*). Therefore in Freudian language, we don't know ourselves because we have so many embedded inner struggles that we are afraid to set free; and as a result we may live in unhealthy denial. Freud's descriptions and work with his own dreams and the dreams of his patients are forays into the paradoxical poetry of the dream. One can be simultaneously seduced and terrified by such poetic imagery. Freud encourages his patients to recognise this restless soul of the unconscious in an effort to help the patient 'cure' themselves. This process of recognition is a practice of care that involves a protracted period of psychoanalysis, where Freud or the Freudian psychoanalyst is 'midwife to the soul' (Bettelheim 1984, p. 36). In this process of psychoanalysis the patient (analysand) can themselves unleash the restlessness of their soul, so that the analyst can draw attention and connection to what has been stifled. The 'unconscious thinking' (Freud 1997, p. 172) of the latent dream content is presented in 'hieroglyphics' whose symbols, says Freud, 'must be translated one by one, into the language of dream-thoughts' (1997, p. 169). 'It would of course be incorrect to attempt to read these symbols in accordance with their values as pictures, instead of in accordance with their meaning as symbols' (1997, pp. 69, 170). From this we can take that the surface depiction of the dream images has a deeper symbolic signification. It may be that we seem to remember a fragment of the detail of something that we feel to be much larger, something that was a consuming part of the whole night. Freud notes that this shows a 'disproportion between dream-contents and dream-thoughts [and] justifies the conclusion that a considerable condensation of psychic material occurs in the formation of dreams' (1997, p. 171). In this way we are 'deprived of access' (1997, p. 171) but because it is within our own psyches, it's also within our own power to reclaim what is lost or hiding in the depths of the soul.

> Nowhere in his writings does Freud gives us a precise definition of the term "soul." I suspect that he chose the term *because* of its inexactitude, its emotional resonance. Its ambiguity speaks for the ambiguity of the psyche itself, which reflects many different, warning levels of consciousness simultaneously.
>
> *(Bettelheim 1984, p. 77)*

These ambiguities of the psyche as manifested in dreams represent some of the dream material that will allow us to access our archetypes in the practical exercises of this chapter. For the remainder of the book I will try to distinguish the soul from the psyche despite their conflation amongst many of my sources. The position I take is that the soul is a deep kernel of the psyche but is not separate from it. The psyche is more encompassing than the soul and includes the entire non-bodily self.

Carl Gustav Jung (1875–1961), the psyche/soul and the archetype

Like Freud, Jung (2002) conflates the psychic centre with the soul, which he says is not regulated from outside (e.g. society) but from within. And it is this interior that we may hide from, therefore hiding from our own souls. 'People will do anything, no matter how absurd, in order to avoid facing their own souls' (Jung 2002, p. 174). Jung notes that the psychic centre also has 'the quality of "eternity" or relative timelessness' (2002, p. 181) and 'is a problem of *all* life' (my emphasis); in this way Jung extends the psychic self into a limitless space and time (2002, p. 200). The unconscious psyche may even 'transcend' and 'surround' the conscious on 'all sides' (2002, p. 215). He suggests another level in the psyche that he calls 'the above conscious', which I include in my diagram, Plate 5 in the colour-plate section at the back of the book (Jung 2002, p. 215). For Jung the unconscious and above conscious content connects backwards and forwards to 'archetypal data' (2002, p. 215). The post-Jungian James Hillman (1979) explains the passage of communication across consciousness to the archetypes in the dream as a 'bridge inward' with one's back to the waking world and facing the dream world (Hillman 1979, p. 6).

The archetypal figures, which I enlarge upon in the following pages, can be aspects of a deep past, and of 'ancestral life' (Jung 2002, p. 214). And, to this backwards and forwards movement I add that the unconscious also moves inwards to the 'physiological states' of the body (Jung 2002, p. 215). These propositions are represented in Plate 5 where there is also a dynamic spatiality outside of the illustrated sphere of consciousness. Therefore in the effort to attain wholeness, we should avoid 'splitting off the unconscious' because Jung warns that this brings 'about an unbearable alienation of instinct. [And] Loss of instinct is the source of endless error and confusion' (Jung 2002, p. 14).

Generally, Jungian psychology presents the psyche in the following way but it's important to note that all three are mobile and tend to overlap: A. the persona/ego – the public mask of the self, the part that is protective of what lies beneath; B. the shadow – the alternative parts of the self, that is the vulnerable and/or neglected part of the self, which has not been allowed to reach potential; C. the anima/animus – the female and male part of the self.

The description and deconstruction of the self by Jung can be helpful in the production of art from dreams because, for every conscious concept there is a 'related psychic association' (Jung et al. 1979, p. 29). The psychic associations take on forms in dreams:

> The images produced in dreams are much more picturesque and vivid than the concepts and experiences that are their waking counterparts. One of the reasons for this is that, in a dream, such concepts can express their

unconscious meaning. In our conscious thoughts, we restrain ourselves within the limits of rational statements – statements that are much less colourful because we have stripped them of most of the psychic associations.

(Jung et al. 1979, p. 29)

The dream image in Plate 6 in the colour-plate section is an example of a dream with blinding psychedelic colour that formed an impenetrable space for the emaciated dream figure already balancing a load on her head.

As I understand Jung, all our archetypes emanate from the persona and its shadow, so one can have a few archetypes that appear dominant in the public face and then there are those that are part of the shadow self. We are not always in touch with both sides; they are not always in sync – and this is also true of the anima/animus, female/male parts of ourselves. Dreams for Jung are a spontaneous self-portrayal in symbolic form and not symptomatic as they also tend to be with Freud. Jung believed the psyche to be a self-regulating organism. He cautioned against blindly ascribing meaning to dream symbols without a clear understanding of one's personal situation. Jung (2002) also said that he approached every dream as a beginner. The dreamer's unconscious is the key to the dream and therefore it is up to that person to bring in associations but if desired an available Jungian analyst/therapist can incorporate myth as appropriate. Understanding archetypes is an important route into Jungian dream theory because archetypes are usually present in some form in all dreams. Archetypal dreams are also referred to as 'mythic dreams' which have a cosmic quality and are generally vivid.

The four primary categories that Jung (1972) gives his archetypes are: Mother; Rebirth; Spirit; Trickster. The *Mother* archetype is also often referred to as the Great Mother, the nurturer, and, in line with the anima and the animus, s/he can be of androgynous gender as well as being both 'good' and 'bad', as the giver s/he can be jealous of what s/he protects. The *Rebirth* archetype is also sometimes represented as a divine child; for example when Jung writes of 'archetypal rebirth' (1972, p. 86), this is a return to the inner child and the true self in its purest form. In recognising this archetype, it may be possible to regain full potential and be open to all possibilities. The *Spirit* archetype is an 'immaterial substance or form of existence which on the highest and most universal level is called "God"' (Jung 1972, p. 86). This spirit archetype may also represent an eternal wisdom. The *Trickster* archetype plays jokes to keeps us from taking ourselves too seriously on the one hand but also to encourage us to consider obscure alternatives and sudden possibilities. However, from these four overarching archetypes, there are an unlimited number/variation which abound in diverse sources, some examples are tabulated alphabetically in Table 2.1.

It is obvious that the self and its psyche are not singular in Jungian language and he points out that to gain unity of an otherwise fragmented self, ancient rites of transformation and renewal may be useful. He defends this approach, saying that if rituals that involved archetypal persona had not worked in the ancestral past, they would have died out (Jung 2002, p. 214). In other words when we

TABLE 2.1 Common Archetypes

Common Archetypes				
Anarchist	Dreamer	Matriarch	Puppet	Spy
Artist	Eternal Boy/ Girl	Mistress	Puritan	Star
Avenger	Evangelist	Monk	Queen	Storyteller
Beggar	Fae /Fairy	Muse	Rebel	Student
Brat	Fool	Mystic	Rescuer	Teacher
Bureaucrat	Gambler	Nature Boy/Girl	Revolutionary	Tempest
Caregiver/taker	God	Navigator	Rock star	Temptress
Chameleon	Goddess	Networker	Saboteur	Thief
Child	Gossip	Nun	Sadist	Tramp
Class Clown	Harlot	Olympian	Sage	Trickster
Clown	Healer	P/Matriarch	Samaritan	Tyrant
Coach	Herald	Passenger	Scarlet Woman	Vampire
Companion	Hermit	Pilgrim	Scholar	Victim
Coward	Historian	Pioneer	Scout	Virgin
Craftsperson	Innovator	Poet	Seducer	Visionary
Crone	Judge	Politician	Seeker	Warrior
Crook	King	Predator	Seer	Wise Woman
Damsel	Knight	Priest/ Priestess	Servant	Witch
Detective	Liberator	Prince	Settler	Wizard
Deviant	Lolita	Princess	Shaman	
Dictator	Lover	Prophet	Sidekick	
Diplomat	Magician	Prostitute	Slave	
Disciple	Martyr	Provocateur	Slut	
Diva	Masochist	Prude	Spoiler	

become stagnated or feel weary and weighed down in this contemporary world of scepticism and speed, it may be useful to renew and refresh ourselves, even using rituals that might seem part of a lost age.

We can get in touch with our unconscious archetypes through symbolic representations in this world. The archetype usually remains in the unconscious and can be accessed in two ways. One is through manifestations in and of the unconscious (for example, dreams), and the other is through myths that we may relate to. The symbols in a myth become archetypal images. Both Freud and Jung used Ancient Greek, Roman and Egyptian mythology to assist in understandings of the unconscious. The archetypes are the qualities of the dream and myth symbols, but they are also qualities of the psyche. Additionally it is important to remember that (our) archetypes are not fixed but in flux. For example, Achilles in Homer's *Iliad* is both the swift-footed and ruthless warrior but also the fiercely loyal friend. 'The archetype consists of both form and energy' (Jung 1972, p. 36) and they are interwoven in our dreams, their frequent ambiguity making them more difficult to recognise.

The Collective Unconscious

Jung's writing on 'first dreams' (the first ones we can recall /remember from childhood) is important when identifying significant archetypes that might reappear during the rest of one's life dreams. It was from his work on first dreams that Jung came to understand the presence and significance of the collective unconscious. First dreams are different to other dreams:

> they contain symbolical images which we also come across in the mental history of mankind. It is worth noting that the dreamer does not need to have any inkling of the existence of such parallels. This peculiarity is characteristic of dreams of the individuation process, where we find the mythological motifs or mythologems I have designated as archetypes. These are to be understood as specific forms and groups of images which occur not only at all times and in all places but also in individual dreams, fantasies, visions, and delusional ideas. Their frequent appearance in individual case material, as well as their universal distribution prove that the human psyche is unique and subjective or personal only in part, and for the rest is collective and objective.
>
> *(Jung 1974, p. 77)*

The archetype of predator in the form of a wolf appeared in the very first dream I recall having as a young child. In the dream I wanted to go from the house where I was sleeping to the hotel where my mother was still working whilst I slept. There was a thorny hedge on the side of the path between the two buildings which is where my predator lay in wait. It remains clear in my consciousness to this day and may have been a recurring dream for its strength to persist. I include an illustration that I made of this childhood dream whilst engaging in dream work in my adult life (see Plate 7 in the colour-plate section).

As we proceed through life into youth, adulthood and older years, we accumulate the joys and woes of the world into our unconscious, for example the joy of love and generosity, and the sorrow of poverty and pain. To this end Jung writes that when we have 'big' dreams, the archetypal imagery in those dreams often comes from the collective unconscious and collective/global concerns more than from the personal. The collective unconscious and its archetypes lie at a deeper level than the personal unconscious (Jung, 1974, p. 77) and are not only related to current concerns and future concerns but also across time into a deep past. This primordial time is something that we will address in the topic of dreamtime and indigenous stories in Chapter 3.

Large archetypal dreams often occur at significant phases in our life. 'They reveal their significance – quite apart from the subjective impression they make – by their plastic form, which often has a poetic force and beauty' (Jung 1974, p. 77). Jung says that these epic dreams make a lasting impression on the waking consciousness but in his experience they are very difficult to interpret. They are filled with rich content imagery which can be used for imaginative arts practice. Jung (1974) writes that in fathoming the dreams it is useful to return to the mythical meaning of the symbols presented through the archetypes.

In this theoretical section of Chapter 2, Freud and Jung's ideas on the soul and psyche are presented with the thoughts of Foucault and Nietzsche. Following Jung we have explored the constitution of the self as part of a universe and into which several archetypes take form across the lifespan. As such Jung's belief in the interplay of the ego and its shadow presents an internal alliance that can be used for personal growth. The exercises which follow in the practical section involve shadow work, mandala and ritual.

Section B: Practical: the unconscious and healing practices – archetypes and shadows

For all of the exercises below it's important for you to centre yourself and be quiet; you can use the mindfulness breathing techniques from Section A of Chapter 1 as well as meditation music to calm your mind and body before embarking on the exercises.

Exercises

Dream shadow work

This first exercise involves tasks to increase your self-knowledge. You will be guided to reflect on any emergence of archetypal forms or figures in the recollection of a recent or prominent dream. An exercise in dialoguing with the archetype includes use of non-dominant and dominant hands in the act of writing down that conversation, and also in the subsequent artwork.

Materials: specific art materials that have fluidity and freedom are recommended, for example charcoal, oil pastel, watercolour, clay.

Before you commence the exercise it might help to see how one of my students (whom I will call Alice), approached and executed this exercise. Alice's examples shown in Figures 2.1, 2.2, and 2.3, and the excerpts from her dream narrative are only a guide; it's important for you to source your own dream image. Also, remember that the textual narrative is *not* what goes into the dream journal when the dreamer awakes, but what is done later as part of the processing. Figure 2.1 is the drawing Alice did first, while Figures 2.2 and 2.3 including the written narrative were developed from the initial dream image recollection.

Alice's accompanying dream narrative explains the presence of a large spider above the bed in a recurring dream. For Alice, in the initial stages of her dreamwork, the spider is a metaphor for entrapment and fear:

> Dangles above my sleep, light legs all stretching to touch me,
> hold, grab and envelope into the darkness,

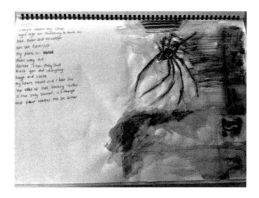

FIGURE 2.1 *Alice's Spider Dream Version 1* (2014), charcoal and wash on art journal paper.
Reproduced in accordance with ethics protocols.

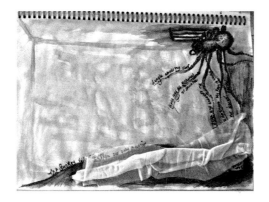

FIGURE 2.2 *Alice's Spider Dream Version 2* (2014), charcoal, pen, paint and fabric, collage
in an art journal.
Reproduced in accordance with ethics protocols.

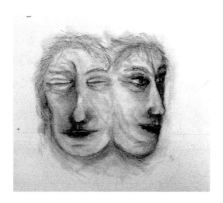

FIGURE 2.3 *Alice's Shadow Self* (2014), charcoal and graphite pencil in an art journal.
Reproduced in accordance with ethics protocols.

my path is veiled, which way out, darker,
I can only just make you out dangling huge and close,
my heart races and I feel sick,
the veil of soft smoky chiffon is the only barrier,
is it through cold fear – wakes me, it's so real.

And Alice's concluding narrative after the image development is as follows:

> From the spider overhead to naked split persona, the mother archetype is
> the one I see often in my dreams; even as male protagonists . . . see myself
> looking back, questioning me; fear of letting go and allowing my true self to
> emerge is evident through my dreams. By this better understanding of the
> inner self – closure on several issues have been resolved. Allowing the nega-
> tive feelings towards my own mother and motherhood leave my psyche with
> a sense of relief which has fallen over me – allowing the inner child to emerge
> and ask for help is a form of letting go of adult control over my creativity – a
> freedom to express more fluidly will be my continuing journey.

At this point it's worth considering the thoughts of Hillman (1979) on animals
in dreams for what might provide additional insight into dreams similar to this one
that Alice had. Hillman reminds us that the animal kingdom is larger than ours and
that to look at animals in dreams is to see them as 'carriers of soul' (1979, p. 148).
Whilst acknowledging the entrapment metaphor of spiders, Hillman contests that
the 'spinning illusion' is 'mandala forming' and that such spider dreams point to a
fear of 'the unconscious force of integration' (1979, p. 149). He says that we should
not diagnose the spider too readily and rather look into our egos where we may
need to accept the synthetic powers of our imagining.

Process

1 Look at the list of archetypes in Table 2.1 and choose one as your dominant
  and one as its shadow (the shadow is usually its opposite). Consult your
  dream journal for clues.
2 Put your hands in front of you on the table and look at them quietly and
  closely; feel them as an extension of your arms, your torso, your heart's core.
3 Which is the dominant hand? Which is the non-dominant?
4 Reflect on these two sides of your whole body for a moment noting their differences (if you feel comfortable, you can close your eyes to do this).
5 Imagine that your dream world lies in your non-dominant side and your
  waking/outer world lies in your dominant side. Reflect upon where you are
  now in your state of consciousness: are you between your two hands/sides
  or firmly in one?
6 Now take your *non-dominant* hand and, choosing a loose or fluid medium,
  make/draw your *dominant archetype* (one that you recognise consciously).

7   Then, when you're finished. Take your *dominant* hand and make/draw your *shadow self*. This will probably be the opposite archetype to the dominant one.

Spend some time reflecting on the influence of the unconscious side on the conscious or of the uncontrolled side on the controlled side. Consider what insights you've discovered from your body – mind and how they might inform your arts practice.

Allow yourself enough time for stages 6 and 7 of this exercise. And if you have time to spare, repeat the whole exercise with other choices from the list of archetypes in Table 2.1.

Inside/outside mask work

This is a slightly different shadow exercise which acknowledges your waking outer self which are visualised as the mask(s) we have to wear, as well as your inner shadow self/ves. The term mask is used simply instead of cover; you do not need to draw a mask shape but if you want to experiment afterwards, you can make your own symbolic masks in different materials or you can purchase blank masks from a craft store and decorate them accordingly.

1   You need four pieces of A3 paper which you join together with adhesive tape, so that two pieces flap over as the two 'fronts' meeting in the centre. Then there are also the two (or four if you want to use the reverse side of the fronts) in the inside lying beside each other. See Figure 2.4.
2   With the two 'fronts' before you and with coloured pastels, quickly cover your dominant side front with a typical mask of emotion that you have to wear at work. And then also quite quickly, cover the other subdominant front with a different 'mask' which you often also need to wear in other social/public situations. Do not use text.
3   Now open out the covers to reveal the blank insides.

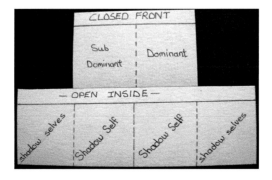

FIGURE 2.4   *Inside/Outside Explanatory Diagram* (2018).

Author's own artwork.

4   You can work across the joined pieces or separate them. Fill the insides with your shadow selves in any way that comes to you; this can be abstract but the symbols must mean specific things to you.

5   Spend some time reflecting on your outside – inside, noting the responses in your body. What do you feel? What do you hear? If there are musical or other sounds for the outside masks, what are these sounds? What instruments are playing? And for the inside, your shadow selves, what music or sounds do you hear, what musical instruments are used? What is the balance between silence and sound? More work will be done on sound in Chapter 6.

Mandala work

The mandala exercise is a good but basic tool. The symmetry of the mandala might help you put various things into a comfortable place. The designing of a personal mandala can be described as representative of your psychic patterns coalescing into a whole. The personal mandala can similarly adopt your most common archetypes and distribute them across your mandala symbolically. Jung suggests that the 'true mandala' is 'gradually built up through (active) imagination' (1974, p. 171) therefore you can take time over this exercise and revise it over a period of months or even years. Jung's magnificent mandala paintings, which can be seen in his *The Red Book: Liber Novus*, took a lifetime of work (Jung 2009).

Materials: paper/card or canvas; paints or oil pastels (to make more permanent mandalas, you can use fabrics and mosaics at a later stage).

1   Have a *square* piece of good quality paper, card or canvas.

2   Take a ruler and lightly draw lines through the centre so that you start off with four equal quadrants and a clear central point.

3   With a maths compass or a round plate draw a circle in the square leaving an even space for a border pattern. See Figure 2.5. You can then draw triangles or circles in the outer rim of the circle towards the corners of the square.

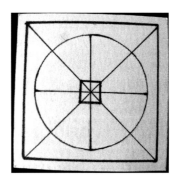

FIGURE 2.5 *Mandala Basic Template Example* (2018).

Author's own work.

4   If you feel inhibited and need a template for your mandala pattern, there are many beautiful mandalas on the internet which you can use as exemplars, but ensure that the visual symbolism is from your own unconscious.

5   Consult your dream journal *or* redo the states of consciousness exercise (in Chapter 1 of this book).

6   Choose a dominant figure or form and a few subdominant ones from the above source(s). Have them visible beside you.

7   You can now transfer your dominant and subdominant selves (your archetypes) into the patterned surface.

8   As you select colours, patterns and shapes, remember that the whole mandala is your 'psychic centre' which, as Jung says, is not to be confused with the ego (1974, p. 173).

9   The mandala is an exercise that need not and perhaps should not be completed in one day. When you think it's complete, put it up somewhere and let it speak to you, what is this representation of your soul saying about who you are?

Ritual and self-knowledge

The exercises 'shadow dream work', 'mask work' and 'mandala work' above should be catalysts for healing in the process of recognising yourself and caring for your self, but this third exercise of 'ritual' can be a culminating one, where all parts can come together in movement through space.

Materials: in this exercise it is your body and props that you'll need for costume and choreography, so the materials depend on how you design your ritual. The example that I provide from a ritual performance I enacted with a class of trainee creative therapists is a type of dance ritual where I am carrying a burden that I relinquish. The materials I included were: music; black hand-beaded netting; black clothing; a large stone.

The ritual exercise can be done alone but it's most useful when you have trusted friends who can silently witness for you. It can be inside or out in nature.

Preparation

•   Consider three circles of your world and your life: 1) your ordinary everyday world; 2) representing lows and falls; 3) a time or moments of renewal.

•   You can map this out on paper first and prepare what props and materials you need for each stage or circle. An example of what I sketched in preparation for a ritual performed for my art therapy group is shown in Figures 2.6, 2.7 and 2.8.

•   It helps to practise because you'll improvise movements and acknowledge what is ordinary, what is low and what is renewal, as you dance or move through the space.

•   It may help to crystallise your choreography if you draw diagrams and make notes as you practise.

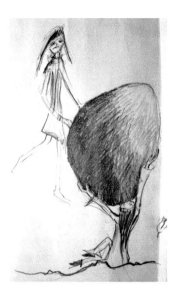

FIGURE 2.6 Kathleen Connellan (2015), *Ordinary, Everyday*, graphite pencil on paper.
Author's own artwork.

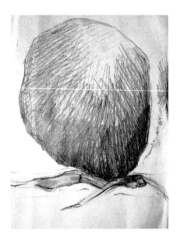

FIGURE 2.7 Kathleen Connellan (2015), *Falling*, graphite pencil on paper.
Author's own artwork.

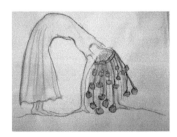

FIGURE 2.8 Kathleen Connellan (2015), *Ritual Performance Preparatory Drawing*, coloured pencil on paper.
Author's own artwork.

- My advice is to keep it simple so that you can be aware of your body and not have to worry about details when you are actually in your performance.
- Some suggestions: you might want to 'burn' or bury something or you may want to preserve something that needs to be retrieved, restored and then framed or displayed.
- This will be an art performance piece for you so you might also want to ask a friend to video it.
- It's a good idea to join in a celebratory meal afterwards.

Conclusion

This chapter has adopted the position that we have a dominant public self and private shadow selves, all of which may be connected to archetypes. It is necessary to wear different masks to function in the social and professional world; however, we also need to be aware of the inner self or selves and what they mean. The Ancients like Socrates offer wisdom on knowing and caring for the self as a daily practice. This philosophy influenced generations of thinkers including Foucault, Nietzsche, Freud and Jung, all of whom are referred to in the chapter. The soul as a core constituent of the self is therefore presented in this chapter as vulnerable and susceptible to being overburdened. The practical section presents healing ways of symbolising all these aspects of the soul-self in art forms, whether in mask work, mandala paintings or performance.

Note

1 The reader who is already familiar with the philosophers referred to might find it incongruous to use Jung and Foucault in the same chapter (or even in the same book), and I hope to address such concerns by embracing post-Jungian openness and also returning to the work of the Ancient Greek philosophers, such as Socrates and Seneca, so often used by Foucault. The comprehensive work by Andrew Samuels is the best resource for readers who are sceptical of Jung's nineteenth-century essentialist and gendered language. Jung's anima/animus is in itself an acknowledgement of complex gendering that is in no way binary. For more on Jung and homophobia see Walker (1991); but for refreshing insights into post Jungian activism see Vaughan (2018) which is a lively interview between Alan Vaughan and Andrew Samuels on Jung.

References

Bettelheim, B. (1984), *Freud and Man's Soul*, Vintage, New York.

Foucault, M. (2005), *The Hermeneutics of the Subject: Lectures at the Collège de France 1981–1982*, trans. G. Burchell, Picador, New York.

Foucault, M. (2010), *The Government of Self and Others: Lectures at the Collège de France 1982–1983*, trans. G. Burchell, Palgrave Macmillan, New York.

Freud, S. (1997), *The Interpretation of Dreams*, trans. A.A. Brill, Wordsworth Classics, Ware.

Giegerich, W. (1991), 'The advent of the guest: shadow integration and the rise of psychology', *Spring: A journal of archetype and culture*, vol. 51, pp. 86–106.

Hillman, J. (1979), *The Dream and the Underworld*, Harper & Row, New York.

Homer (2003), *The Iliad*, trans. E.V. Rieu, Penguin Books, London.

Jung, C.G. (1972), *Four Archetypes: Mother, rebirth, spirit, trickster*, trans. R.F.C. Hull, Routledge & Kegan Paul, London.

Jung, C.G. (1974), *Dreams*, trans. R.F.C. Hull, Princeton University Press, Princeton, NJ.

Jung, C.G., von Franz, M.L., Henderson, J.L., Jacobi, J. and Jaffé, A. (1979), *Man and His Symbols*, Picador, New York.

Jung, C.G. (2002), *Dreams*, trans. R.F.C. Hull, Routledge, London.

Jung, C.G. (2009), *The Red Book: Liber Novus*, trans. M. Kyburz, J. Peck and S. Shamdasani, Norton & Company, London.

Nietzsche, F. (1976), *The Portable Nietzsche*, trans. W Kaufmann, Penguin, Harmondsworth.

Vaughan, A.G. (2018), 'A conversation between like-minded colleagues and friends: Alan Vaughan and Andrew Samuels', *Jung Journal*, vol. 12, no. 2, pp. 118–137.

Walker, M. (1991), 'Jung and homophobia', *Spring: A journal of archetype and culture*, vol. 51, pp. 55–71.

3

BELONGING

Dreaming and place

Introduction

Dreams almost always have a setting; they take place 'somewhere'. That place is often also quite recognisable even if the space is uncanny. The English translation (uncanny) of the German word *unheimliche*, which is literally translated as 'unhomely', fails to capture the understanding that Freud developed of the uncanny; namely not simply as something familiar rendered unfamiliar, but more as something that was once 'safe', now becoming 'unsafe'. The places in nocturnal dreams are unsettling because they disturb the presumed security of the real. In contrast, daytime reveries or daydreams can be used to shape wonder-filled images of belonging. This chapter will address 'being' and 'longing' and it will do so with a variety of dream explorations into places of belonging.

The structure of the chapter is divided into theory and practice, situating the conscious theorisation of place in Section A and the practical dream exercises in Section B. Section A begins with excerpts from dream theory that focus on place in dreams and in the imagination. It also includes explanations of the balance between the real (functional everyday) and the ideal (desired) in constructing places of belonging. This is done through the categories of indigenous place, landscape and metaphorical space. Metaphorical space includes a discussion of *temenos* which is an ideal and spiritually centred space, one that will be taken further in the practical exercises that form Section B of this chapter. To avoid slippage between the terms 'place' and 'space', I use the term 'space' as something that we can shape ourselves, and 'place' as an already established locale. Section A prepares the reader for exercises and reflections on ancestral and indigenous connections to place as a means of developing understandings of home. These conscious creations of home and places of belonging will build upon the previous chapters' information on self-knowledge and self-doubt by situating the self in particular environments which may add to, or detract from, feeling safe and at home. Section B draws from the unconscious and the preconscious. First, it focusses on the unconscious dreams and dream images of spaces and places that have emerged and may yet emerge from nocturnal dream journaling. Second, there are additional exercises on finding healing places and designing safe therapeutic spaces for yourself in both your mind and in your homes.

Section A: Theory: conscious reflections on belonging

The dream place

In the dream there is an awareness of place, a consciousness of the type of space one is in, even though the dream is in the realm of the unconscious. Jung explains the typical form of what he calls an 'average' dream, and the importance of place is distinct in this; Jung's sequential dream phases are summarised below (2002, pp. 82, 83):

A   – Statement of place:

1   Details about the protagonist (dreamer). E.g. I was in a house with my friend X [and] at the top of the stairs Mrs T bumped into X.
2   Further details about the protagonist. E.g. I was in a dress suit and X was in pyjamas.

B   – Development of action:

1   Further details about the plot, e.g. what happened next, therefore some indication of time sequence. E.g. 'Mrs. T seemed to be very agitated and wanted to tell us something but struggled to speak.'
2   Further complication and tension develops in the plot.

C   – Culmination:

1   Decisive occurrence or complete change. E.g. Suddenly Mrs T's face contorted and she fell down the stairs.

D   – Solution/result (Jung says this final phase is often lacking in dreams):

1   Evidence of the protagonist/dreamer seeking solution.
2   A new reflectiveness after the preceding confusion.
    E.g. We rushed down the stairs but when we got there Mrs T had disappeared. My friend X said she'd probably gone to hospital and we should visit her.

In this Jungian dream sequence there are two descriptors of place that set the scene and the action (1) the house and (2) the stairs. Both facilitate development of the dream narrative but also provide symbolic spatial indicators for the dreamer. Relationships are represented and challenged in a space, action occurs through space and resolution happens in another place. The psycho-physical environment provides three-dimensional spatiality to the dream narrative.

This conjunction between the physical person, the place one is in and the symbolic or psychic space has inspired many artists, writers and architects. A well-known example from visual art is Giorgio de Chirico's 1914 oil painting *Mystery and Melancholy of a Street*. This surreal painting, which can be found easily on the internet, shows a lonely street with deep arches in vanishing perspective, a silhouetted child running with a hoop and a long figurative shadow approaching. The aura is immediately uncertain, the perspective is inaccurate and the colours are unnatural. All this is compounded by the strange night ambience of yellowed orange, blue and deep browns. Then it is also worth looking at examples of Martinus Escher's 1950s lithographs with impossibly dense interiors and open stairways leading both everywhere and nowhere. In poetry, Edgar Allan Poe's nineteenth-century short story 'The Fall of the House of Usher' is yet another uncanny interior filled with the unknown. In such dreamscape designs, the formal structures of architectural and spatial accuracy are deliberately out of balance thus illustrating the madness in an uncontrolled unconscious.

However, whilst artists, poets and musicians can distort and destroy the sane structures of balanced space, architects cannot. Nonetheless, despite having to design buildings that are safe, some architects also want to create dreams spaces and to do this the visible reassurances of load-bearing structures are rendered invisible. They are there but are either hidden or disguised, thereby resulting in a space that occupants are unsure of. For example, the architect Peter Eisenman achieves a 'schizographic condition' (Vidler 1992, p. 143) in order to achieve a space that is real but 'disturbingly disturbed' (1992, p. 143). Entering such architectural spaces that challenge the expected flow and structure of the built space can feel like entering a dreamscape. Eisenman's designs resist having a centre which is also the repression of a stable base, even the denial of a visible heart of a space (like the symbolic fireplace in the home). When real built spaces have no such centre, each interior axis dissolves into, or is broken by another axis (Vidler 1992, p. 143).

These interruptions fracture conscious expectations of 'reality' and provide analogies and possibilities for dream spaces. In the dream one is never comfortably at home, or centred, or sure of where one is or where one should go; these spatial questions are deeply psychic. The feeling of being in the 'right' place is counterbalanced by a longing for what is missing. And whilst the uncanny ambiguous dream space provides inspiration for exciting and unpredictable architecture, such spaces can also be daunting. For example, I have written elsewhere about the psychic life of white spaces, where walls dissolve into an apparently free flowing space but where the self is thus rendered peculiarly vulnerable and watched (Connellan 2013).

Indigenous place

Another dimension to place and space are the spiritual aspects. In a recent project, I collaborated with colleagues[1] in conducting research in a mother – baby mental health unit. The unit is a new architectural design on an old site that has a historic mortuary building. This mortuary building has beautiful exposed blue-stone blocks in a neo-Gothic style. The architects wanted to adapt and incorporate the mortuary as the main entrance for the unit. This design was strongly opposed by the community who voiced concern for the spirits of those who had passed and the families of those who remained. Indeed Indigenous Australians requested that the space be left to house its ancestral spirits (interview data). This wish was honoured.

Place and country are key to Indigenous Australian dreaming. Indigenous Australian dreaming and dreamtime is known as *tjurkurrpa*, which is intrinsically connected to the land; any images that contain *tjurkurrpa* are coded to prevent illegitimate sharing of sacred knowledges. I cannot speak for Indigenous Australians but their voices should be heard. One such voice sings out through her dream sharing the poignancy and pain of Indigenous place.

> In this dream, a daytime dream, I was walking – walking with a big mob of people to the place where my granddaughters would grow. And as we walked I could hear sounds of laughing, singing, sadness, crying. Big mobs of people together walking to some place – into the future. I asked "Where are we going?" and the answer came "To a place." I asked "How will we know that place?" and the answer came "We'll know"! We came to a place, the place? This place!
>
> *(Atkinson 2002, p. 1)*

Connection to place is deeply spiritual with certain areas marked as sacred. The spirit of place is the spirit of ancestors, and something seemingly inanimate like a rock can hold a millennium of secrets. Recently my husband and I travelled to the Flinders Ranges in South Australia for a few days. The majesty of those landscapes are filled with a dreaming that is palpable; it hangs in the air and whispers from the stones, red earth and knuckled mountain tops. In personal conversations with Indigenous Australians, I was told that the knuckles are those of the original owners of the land, the *Adnyamathanha*, who are the Aboriginal people of the northern Flinders Ranges. The South Australian Department of Environment (2018) translates *Adnyamathanha* as 'hills' or 'rock people' incorporating the traditional groups in the Flinders Ranges.

Nici Cumpston, an Adelaide artist and curator of Indigenous art at the Art Gallery of South Australia, is from the *Barkindji* people, associated with the River Murray. This great river flows from the northern regions of the Australian continent all the way down to the Southern Ocean. 'We are the people of the river', Cumpston said in a talk 'On her artistic practice and the personal and historical stories behind her work in *Troubled Waters*' at the Samstag Museum of Art in Adelaide, in May 2017 during National Reconciliation Week. *Ringbarked II* (Plate 8 in the colour-plate section at the back of the book) is one of Cumpston's hand-painted photographs of dead trees on the banks of the River Murray. The site is layered with Aboriginal archaeology which must yet be studied in full. When colonial settlers came to the River-land, they manipulated the great river Murray to alter its flow and expand its banks for farm irrigation. On one occasion when the water was drained back to its original water level, the site with dead trees was exposed. 'Dead in the water', says Cumpston, as her trees sigh with silent immortal pain behind her on the gallery wall. Cumpston had always felt a connection to that part of the river but did not know why because her people are from much farther away in the north-eastern part of the country close to the Darling River. However, subsequently consulting with Aboriginal Elders in that region, she discovered that the exposed banks, trees, roots and rocks showed markings of her own people who, like others, came to meet and camp (*larundel*) in that place a long time ago.

The pain of those old trees now dead, the tragedy of the great river once free flowing and flooding the plains, but now dammed and threatened, are the voices of Cumpston's ancestors as they call out in warning for a country under the siege of apparent progress. The incredible age of Indigenous country and custom speaks a language through dreamtime.

To walk in that country and witness its natural grandeur from the heights of the ranges to the depths of the creeks and gorges is to be in the presence of something outside of material reality. Within the context of dreaming, healing and imaginary arts practice, the Flinders and the Riverland are spiritual places. One often just wants to be silent and still in such a place; to hear, sense and feel the voices of nature, and perhaps, if one is of Indigenous heritage, the voices of ancestral spirits.

Ancestral places are crucial for continued communication with past, present and future for many indigenous peoples on this planet. I do not use the term 'ancestral' lightly and am aware that Bachelard (1994, p. 188) considers the danger of using it 'lazily'. We are all indigenous to some place, and it is likely that we have been to a place which we think is for the first time, but from the moment we arrive there is a deep feeling of belonging and kinship, indeed it is a strangely comforting feeling of 'home'. It is more than *déjà vu*. I felt this when I visited my father's county in Ireland, I went to his grave for the first time in a countryside where (as the song goes) 'the dark mountains of Mourne run down to the sea'. (See Plate 9 in the colour-plate section.)

The sloping, undulating and impossibly green landscape with its historic farmhouses is home to familiarly featured faces. Being in that place helped me recognise a previously uncertain longing. Along with Simon Schama (1995), I acknowledge that it is only humans who can scape the land. However, despite the cruelty invoked upon some of nature's most beautiful spaces, as humans we inhabit this land for better or worse, and the memories, mysteries and dreams that are in it are a part of our intrinsic longings. All these dreams can be used both creatively and constructively. For example in times of grief and loss, people often mark the landscape with a sign of lost loved ones as a place to return to for healing. These signs can be as temporary as flowers attached to a wooden post by the roadside, or more permanent like an inscribed bench.

Metaphorical space

Interiors

In this final part of Section A, we now shift to a more interior understanding of place and space. In Gaston Bachelard's classic work *Poetics of Space* (1994), his feeling of an old home and refuge that might only survive in memory is retrieved in minute and poetic detail. The spaces he writes about include the interior of drawers and closets, the intimacy of corners, and the dialectics of the outside and inside. Bachelard draws on the Bohemian-Austrian poet Rainer Maria Rilke's *Fragments from an Intimate Diary* and others for inspiration and material. There is an occasion when Rilke and friends were travelling alone and on foot 'one very dark night' when they perceived 'the lighted casement of a distant hut, the hut that stands quite alone on the horizon' (Bachelard 1994, p. 36). This then becomes a symbol of vigil, of refuge and of intimacy, but the darker side is that a house which stands alone on a horizon has many besieging forces. Bachelard seems to acknowledge that these are also forces of the mind. Engaging with the poetry, he writes, 'This house, as I see it, is a sort of airy structure that moves about on the breath of time. It really is open to the wind of another time. It seems as though it could greet us every day of our lives in order to give confidence in life' (1994, p. 54). And moving deep into the depths of the house's internal enclosures, Bachelard reminds us of the depths in drawers and cupboards that might not be frequently opened and may even be locked 'like a heart that confides in no one, the key is not on the door' (1994, p. 79).

The symbolic depth of intimate spaces like deep drawers, wardrobes and closets are akin to our unconscious. Keys to these interiors of the unconscious are offered through the visual pathways of dreams, but still the portal of consciousness slams shut upon that imagery when wakefulness descends. The keeper of this unconscious treasure trove is indeed the self but this self needs to be prepared to unlock the mysteries of space and place. Metaphors of cupboards, small rooms and vessels provide possibilities for opening and seeing into the depths of our internal psyche; but the cavernous unconscious is frequently contained in seemingly inaccessible dream form. It is therefore most helpful to allow the body's psyche and not just the mind's psyche to enter those spaces. Yi-Fu Tuan (1977) enlarges upon locational points in space and writes that it is not until the human being is aware of those points that the space can be experienced fully with the body. According to Tuan (1977) the body is always in space but spaces are divided by locational points. The position of the human body in a space, even if it is a dream space, is crucial to the experience of that space. For example is one sitting, or standing, lying or crouched? Tuan notes that 'standing' in a space implies 'achievement' and 'order' (Tuan 1977, p. 15). The direction one is facing or looking towards is also significant, raising questions of what is behind sight and what is ahead. Thinking in a space, creates distance according to Tuan (1977, p. 146) both in the sense of giving breath to the space but also in creating a mental distance to objectify the space. Dreaming in a space may alternatively create a closeness as less critique is involved. The conflict between thoughts which are generally subject to greater control, and dreams which have more freedom, are important considerations when shaping spaces that we can spiritually, emotionally and rationally 'be' at home in.

Despite the compunction to let our spiritual self roam in and out of ideal and imagined interiors, it might help to order to those spaces which house our thoughts and dream images. In such an endeavour to bring order to apparent disorder, Bachelard writes that we should consider the connecting themes of the assumed 'stability' of the house and 're-imagine its reality' adding that 'to distinguish all these images would be to describe the soul of the house; it would mean developing a veritable psychology of the house' (Bachelard 1994, p. 17).

Two leading questions that can be asked of this house in which we dream and think are: 'What are its dominant lines?' And, 'what are its forms?' The lines of a house are the basis for its ensuing forms. The nineteenth-century architecture and art critic John Ruskin called for a harmony of formal aspects (lines, spaces, textures, colours) to ensure that the space has a vital spirit:

> It is not enough that is has the Form, if it have not also the power and life. It is not enough that it has the Power, if it have not the form . . . it is not one nor another that produces it but their union in certain measures . . .
>
> *(Ruskin 2007, pp. 153, 154)*

Bachelard writes that 'a house is imaged as a vertical being. It rises upward' (1994, p. 17). Within this verticality, he distinguishes between the cellar and the attic. Bachelard's spaces belong to a specific era but also to European winters. Houses in more southern regions can sprawl horizontally, with long verandas or covered patios to shade the sun. Whatever the design, the interior of a domestic home which is the private space of our personal lives is indeed 'a concentrated being' and a space that 'appeals to our consciousness of centrality' (Bachelard 1994, p. 17). Both the home that is bathed in the sun of the south with its lines that stretch out and along, and the home clothed in the shade of the north, have their dreamy depths. These need not be the literal depths of a cellar, but the metaphorical depths of where we feel mystery and promise and where we might also feel safe and beautifully at home. And with the security of depth there also needs to be the breath of sufficient height; the words of a Medieval poet Edward Matchett echo this intention:

> Let us make a thing of beauty that long may live when we are gone; Let us make a thing of beauty that hungry souls may feast upon; whether it be in

wood or marble, music, art or poetry, let us make a thing of beauty to help set man's bound spirit free.

(Matchett, cited by Painton 1992, p. 8)

Temenos

'Temenos' is a Greek word meaning sacred place or precinct. It was incorporated into the English language in the 1700s and has had peaks and troughs of usage over the years, according to the *Collins English Dictionary*'s online recorded usage graph. I hope to resurrect this special word not only as a term that has no adequate translation but as an accurate descriptor of a space that we can isolate and shape for ourselves. The Greek root *temnō* from the verb *temnein* means to cut off (*Oxford English Dictionary*); therefore we can carve out a space that is special, sacred and private, and over time we can refurnish or redecorate this space as our spiritual and psychological requirements demand.

Finding, setting and maintaining a temenos is crucial for engaging with the unconscious but as much as this might be a safe space it also takes courage to go there and remain for the necessary amount of time. Jung writes of the 'insuperable desire to run away from the unconscious' and yet the 'relief' experienced when a 'protected temenos' is 'established', 'a taboo area where he will be able to meet the unconscious' (2002, p. 127). Jung reminds us of how ancient cities were founded and protected by carefully choosing an 'inviolable' site (Jung 2002, p. 127). Such ancient cities provided sanctuary just as many churches have provided immunity to persecuted people, and today political embassies can do the same. Historically, the castle (with its own chapel), or the city walls would be surrounded by a moat of deep water to ensure safety from onslaught. Metaphorically it is one's own soul that needs that security and calming, because fears, threats and distractions come in and out if the temenos is not sufficiently set for spiritual seclusion. This metaphorical castle-like temenos is a space where unity can be experienced so that disparate parts merge into one (Jung 2002, p. 156).

A personal temenos need not be an entire home (castle-temenos), it can be a single room, or even a corner space. Bachelard (1994) imbues corners with deep simplicity. The corner has the properties of a safe haven and offers a space where one can be still. Once we have designated that space of stillness, an 'imaginary room rises up around our bodies' (Bachelard, 1994, p. 137). This corner space can be a wonderful temenos in that it 'becomes the chamber of our being' (Bachelard, 1994, p. 138).

Temenos can also be an outside space like a garden, but it needs to be enclosed and have a focus such as a fountain or stream (Jung 2002, p. 194). The sound of running water offers reassuring music whilst its dance catches light and shadow. The flow of water can also fill deep wells within us. Bachelard writes that water 'swallows the shadows' (1983, p. 54). This does not mean that shadows are negative; they have their own cooling, calming potential for contributing to temenos. Tanizaki's 1977 book *In Praise of Shadows* advocates simple, still and shadowed spaces. It is the fall of shadows that create the spaces and the play of those shadows that bring light and life.

Not all spaces in shadow or light are conducive to the creation of a positive temenos, and one can be misled by desiring to return to spaces and places that are unhealthy for our psyche. A subject I am not dealing with in this book is Freud's sexual interpretation of dream spaces (Freud 2010); there are multiple references to interior spaces into which one ventures as a regression to the womb. To this end, Jung (2002, p. 208) writes that returning to the mother's womb as temenos in Freudian theory can be unhealthy.

Faithful to his theory of dreams as wish fulfilment, Freud's own dreams are analysed and several reveal his longing to go to the city of Rome. In one dream, Freud stood on top of a hill and looked at Rome 'shrouded in mist'; analysing this material Freud acknowledges 'the promised land seen from afar' (Freud 2010, p. 216). It is important to stay with the image because places both longed for and dreamed of can disappear 'when fixed in words' (Calvino 1974, p. 87) which is why it is crucial to reconstruct the vision into temenos through art. As with Freud (2010) and Calvino (1974), the longed for place may seem distant or even imaginary like a city in the sky suspended in an ethereal silken web (Calvino 1974, p. 75). Wherever and whatever it is, once reached, that place of temenos can be creatively shaped by your own weaving of waters, valleys and hills.

We now move to Section B which requires working with material from your dreams and dreaming to help create your own personal temenos as a healing place and space.

Section B: Practical: the unconscious and healing practices

Dreaming and place: Joan's dream

This section begins with an example from Joan's dream journal (see Plate 10 in the colour plate section) with my own commentary. This is followed with the first exercise that you can do from your own dream resources.

The dream image is clearly situated in the corner of a pink and purple room. Purple is a colour that recurs in Joan's dream images. The thickness of the wall is distinct but not enclosing on account of the open doorway to the right. An idyllic beachscape lies right outside with a stepped path leading directly down onto the sand. But the dreamer who has an androgynous clown persona is seated at a dressing table before an ornately framed mirror. The reflection is not of the 'clown' but of what appears to be a young woman with a kind face who reaches out of the mirror space to touch the hand of the 'clown'. The young woman is also ambiguously part of the exterior. The contrast between the interior and exterior places is exaggerated as if there is a separation between nature and the freedom it brings. However, Joan did not comment on this in her dream work; what was most profound for Joan was the spatial interruption that the mirror reflection brought. She wrote, 'I felt that I needed to connect with my "wise protector", who has lovingly been with me since childhood, supporting me, protecting me, loving me'. The manifest content of this dream space shows two primary place settings (room and beach) and two primary space settings (self and other). The latent content is the potential movement between these places and spaces and the obstacles that prevent this. During the movement between and around the obvious manifest content of the primary places and spaces, the secondary spatiality of other deeper layers of psychic space may be accessed. The psychic spatiality of the dream is heightened with complementary colours that intensify each other (e.g. purple and yellow are opposites on the colour wheel). The room is elevated and the beach is both below and beyond. There are several binaries in the dream, but it is what lies between them that provide the tension and questions for the dreamer. Some of these questions may be: Should I leave my secure space and venture forth? Should I listen to what my protector is saying? What part of my self is the figure seen only from the back?

Exercises

Your place dream

Materials: This exercise can be made in two dimensions (2-D), flat or semi-raised/relief, or in three dimensions (3-D), for example a box or a sand-scape. For flat work, you need crayons, paints, pencils and paper or card; for relief work you need craft glue (a glue gun is very useful for balsa wood), scissors, card and a range of small objects/images; for 3-D you can make a box out of card or balsa wood or collect sea sand and create a landscape space on an old baking tray with any objects that you need such as shells, stones, artificial or real flowers, wooden or plastic animals and figures. You might feel inspired to make your own little figures with materials of your choosing. Whatever you choose to make, I suggest you take a photo of it afterwards for your records and continued dream work.

1   Recall a recent dream place or a mythical place; refer to your visual dream journal.
2   Draw/build this space empty of inhabitants.

   2-D:

   • Draw people/creatures on separate paper and cut them out. If you don't want to draw them, just draw stick figures and then add curved lines around the 'sticks' so you have a thicker outlined form to cut out. All you really need are silhouettes of figure shapes.
   • Draw furniture shapes and don't worry about perspective and accuracy, just get the basic shape outline and cut them out so they are loose. If you prefer you can cut out basic shapes from internet images or traced from magazines but at this stage they should be uncoloured.

- Now add colour as you recall it from your dream. Add the colour both to the space (walls, floors, ceilings) and to the shapes of figures and furniture.
- You might also want or need to draw in some line detail inside the loose shapes to emphasise clothing items if they require this (e.g. large buttons or pockets) and a table mat for a table or a cushion for a chair.
- When you're satisfied that the colour and detail represent your dream as closely as possible, arrange the forms and figures in your dream space.
- Move the figures around as necessary and, according to your dream narrative, let the figures speak if required, but pay particular attention to how and where they move (or don't move) in the dream space.
- Consider the totality of what you've captured in your dream place reconstruction – was there any significant sound? If so, do you need to accompany your dream construction with a particular song or sounds?

3-D:

- Follow all the steps for 2–D but build the figures and forms out of cardboard, balsa wood, modelling clay or materials of your choice.
- If you are using found objects, these will already have colour and detail so be sure to select those that match your dream content and have symbolic meaning that resonate with your dream place and space.

3   Reflection once the dream place with its spaces is 'completed':

- Pay attention to the distance between objects or interiors and exteriors.
- Consider the significance of the boundary wall's or structures.
- Consider the significance of windows/doors/openings.
- Consider the significance of colour and light.
- Listen to the sounds or to the silence in your dream construction.
- Reflect on your self, your psyche and the persona presented in the dream places and spaces.

Guided meditation exercise: a special gift to yourself

Follow these steps by reading through them first; there is not a lot to remember but it is best that you are not reading the steps whilst meditating. If other noisy or interfering thoughts intrude upon your meditative journey, don't fight them, just notice them, but don't engage with them; they will come and go just like the breezes in the air – *stay in your breath* and it will take your spirit away to a place of peace.

1   Ensure that you have a quiet, comfortable and private space to be with yourself.
2   Sit somewhere so that your feet reach the ground and your back and neck are supported.
3   Become aware of your breath.

4   Take a deep breath through your nasal passages if possible and, close your eyes or softly focus on 'nothing'.

5   With your inner eye watch and feel your breath going in and down as a life-giving force of newness and freshness.

6   Breathe out slowly, breathing out all the old staleness (again using your nasal passages if possible).

7   Continue breathing in newness and breathing out staleness; let your breath be natural and relaxed.

8   Whilst doing this take yourself on a journey, guide yourself on the wings of an angel, on a magic carpet or just flying up and away as light as the spirit of your new breath.

9   Fly as high as the clouds and then through and above them.

10 When you are high above the world, look down on it (all the time breathing naturally and being aware that your breath is your life giving force).

11 Looking down, see yourself as a small dot in that country, in that town (or farm or wherever it is your body is really sitting), notice the rooftops, the trees, rivers, roads and mountains that surround your home place, and looking around notice neighbouring and distant countries across oceans, each with their rivers, mountains, forests and deserts.

12 Then return to the small dot that is you, and notice the house and room your body is sitting in, the chair or sofa; look down on your self sitting there quietly.

13 Then return your visionary eye to the surrounding landscape and find/select a beautiful place for yourself; it might be beside the sea, on the edge of a forest, on a mountain slope, in a little village or in an apartment with a view across a glittering city stretching out to distant hills or plains.

14 Once you have found your special place, fly down to it and into its interior.

15 This is your ideal space; furnish and decorate it simply and beautifully with all that is good for your soul. It might be half inside and half outside incorporating a garden.

16 Settle into that beautiful peaceful space where all that is wonderful is miraculously there.

17 Just be in that space, loving it and loving yourself.

18 Stay as long as you need to.

When you are ready, take a deep breath and on the slow exhale, wriggle your fingers and toes, perhaps stretch a little whilst opening your eyes, returning to the here and now. Have a drink of water.

Designing your own temenos

Now that you know what your ideal and longed for space is, just having returned from it, the aim is to re-create as much as possible of that space's affect, texture and ambience for yourself in reality. There will be practical and budget constraints, but look at these as opportunities for creativity rather than obstacles.

1   Choose a favourite pen or pencil and, on a piece of art paper or in an art journal, make a short list of essential things that your temenos requires.

2   Focus on the elements of air, water, earth and fire and align them with the temenos properties of:

- Air = fresh air; natural light; beautiful shadows and reflections; cool breezes lightly caressing your skin; scents of the season carried with the breeze; light blues; pale greens and whites.
- Water = soothing; musical sounds; clean and bright; cooling; quenching; dancing with the air, fish, birds, water lilies, reeds; all the blues and greens in the colour spectrum.
- Earth = groundedness; ochres (colours of red, white and yellow); stones speckled, rough and smooth; grasses, flowers and plants. Scents of nature's herbs and blossoms. All the hues and tones of nature's rooted abundance. The soft or spiky textures of thick grass, the smoothness of spun silk, the lumpiness of muddy earth.
- Fire = warmth; glow; light in shadows. Golden colours of the sun.

3   Return to your list and, with coloured pencils, add shaded blocks of colours and textures that are important beside each item or detail that you would like in your temenos.

4   Decide where you can realistically create a little temenos for yourself. It might be that this exercise is an inspiration to change an entire room or home to align with your need for a place of peace; but start small and try to have one space in your home that is very special, like an island for your spirit.

5   All you might need is a candle, a large but beautiful cushion, a bowl of flowers, some essential oils and soft music. Or, a favourite chair, a view out of the window onto your garden (which you might want to do a little work in to adjust what you see, possibly a bird bath, a pond, a water feature and a variety of plants that can move in the breeze). These are all personal choices but be guided by your dreams and especially by the place you flew to in your meditation journey.

6   Boundaries are important for your temenos. It might be that you need to make or purchase a light folding screen to partition a section of a room for your time in temenos. It may also be important to create a threshold so that there is a gentle path in and out of your temenos, a spatial boundary. Setting up the boundary is also setting up the time for yourself, you may want to commence and close your time in temenos with the sound of a Buddhist gong. Buddhist singing bowls can be purchased for this and the sounds are beautifully cleansing. You might just want to have a little hand bell that you ring gently. It is very important to draw on your preconscious prompts so that they tell you what is needed. It might just be silence; a very beautiful thing.

7   Complete your list, and set a time aside to make your temenos. When you do, do it with love and generosity to yourself; you deserve it.

In setting up your personal temenos, it might help to refer to the salutogenic approach to design for well-being. Using this approach developed by Aaron Antonovsky (1996) in the early twentieth century, the person has a real relationship with the space and everything in it. There is also the very helpful Planetree approach to health care that focuses on natural light and fresh air (Stichler 2008), and the popular Feng Shui approach that offers advice on the flow of energy in your space (Shurety 1997). The significance of the objects in your space is addressed in Chapter 5 but consider that all the things you select in the space are somehow a part of you or that they can offer you potential for growth and individuation.

Conclusion

In summary, place in dreams provides a crucial context and setting, even when that place might change dramatically in a single dream. The built space of the dream can also be a metaphoric search for home but as Bachelard (1994) writes of the mollusc, who has a shell for a home and whose motto must be: 'one must live to build one's house, and not build one's house to live in' (1994, p. 106). It is therefore an ongoing dynamic. We can learn much from the natural world's exquisite nests and extraordinary coral enclosures; inspirational images can be found in Arndt (2014).

Our family histories also inhabit our sensory memory so using the body's psyche can help contribute to the necessary ingredients for creating a temenos. As stated at the beginning of this chapter, being and longing are joined. To experience a space ontologically is to belong there. This chapter on dreaming and place has stretched across poetry and the imagination providing material and inspiration for the creation of spaces of safety and of peace. Sometimes it just takes one gentle step across the threshold of the ordinary into the extraordinary. This is both the deep space of contemplation and a personalised place that reflects the soul.

Note

1 Clemence Due, Adelaide University, Adelaide; Damien W. Riggs, Flinders University, Adelaide; Clare Bartholomaeus, Flinders University, Adelaide. We have a forthcoming book based on this work: K. Connellan, C. Due, D.W. Riggs and C. Bartholomaeus, *Home and Away: Mothers and babies in institutional spaces,* in the Lexington book series for Critical Perspectives on the Psychology of Sexuality, Gender, and Queer Studies, edited by A.L. Jones, D.W. Riggs and R. Stringer.

References

Antonovsky, A. (1996), 'The salutogenic model as a theory to guide health promotion', *Health Promotion International*, vol. 11, no. 1, pp. 11–18.
Arndt, I. (2014), *Animal Architecture*, Abrams & Chronicle, London.

Atkinson, J. (2002), *Trauma Trails, Recreating Song Lines: The transgenerational effects of trauma in Indigenous Australia*, Spinifex Press, Melbourne.

Bachelard, G. (1983), *Water and Dreams: An essay on the imagination of matter*, trans. E.R. Farrell, Pegasus, Dallas.

Bachelard, G. (1994), *The Poetics of Space: The classic look at how we experience intimate places*, trans. M Jolas, Beacon, Boston, Mass.

Calvino, I. (1974), *Invisible Cities*, trans. W. Weaver, Harcourt Brace Jovanovich, New York.

Collins English Dictionary, viewed 1 June 2018, www.collinsdictionary.com/dictionary/english/temenos.

Connellan, K. (2013), 'The psychic life of white: power and space', *Organisation Studies*, vol. 34, no. 10, pp. 1529–1549.

Freud, S. (2010), *The Interpretation of Dreams*, trans. J. Strachey, Basic Books, New York.

Jung, C.G. (2002), *Dreams*, trans. R.F.C. Hull, Routledge, London.

Oxford English Dictionary, viewed 1 June 2018, *https://en.oxforddictionaries.com/definition/temenos*.

Painton, C. (1992), *Rose Windows*, Thames & Hudson, London.

Ruskin, J. (2007), *The Stones of Venice: Volume 11, The Sea Stories*, illustrated edition, Cosimos Classics, New York.

Schama, S. (1995), *Landscape and Memory*, HarperCollins, London.

Shurety, S. (1997), *Feng Shui for the Home*, Rider, London.

South Australian Department of Environment 2018, 'Aboriginal culture and heritage', viewed 16 July 2016, www.environment.sa.gov.au/parks/Visiting/aboriginal-culture-and-heritage

Stichler, J.F. (2008), 'Healing by design', *Journal of Nursing Administration*, vol. 38, no. 12, pp. 505–509.

Tanizaki, J. (1977), *In Praise of Shadows*, trans. T.J. Harper and E.G. Seidensticker, Leete's Island Books, Sedgwick.

Tuan, Y.F. (1977), *Space and Place: The perspective of experience*, University of Minnesota Press, Minneapolis.

Vidler, A. (1992), *The Architectural Uncanny: Essays in the modern unhomely*, MIT Press, Cambridge.

4

MOVEMENT DREAMS

Escaping and returning

Introduction

This chapter delves into different types of bodily movement in dreams and how these might be captured or represented in imaginative arts practice. Therefore developing the previous chapter's focus on places and spaces, the body *and* its psyche now enter into space as a symbol in flux. The conditions of and restrictions to the movement of this body are elaborated upon using sources from dream theories as wells as Symbolist and Romanticist philosophies.

Movement dreams incorporate paralysis in dreams; this is 'non'-movement or the frustrated and often terrifying inability to move in a dream narrative. Therefore this chapter substitutes 'fight' with 'fright' (frozen movement) because combat is not a specific focus of the chapter. The 'fight/flight' psychophysiological response to heighted anxiety was first conceptualised by Walter Cannon (1914) with 'freeze' joining these responses more recently (Siegal 2010). The subtitle of this chapter, 'escaping and returning' points to how a dream might be communicating flight and a subsequent return. Additionally, the context: stairs, cars, trains, planes, roads, passages; and elements: air, water, earth, fire, for flight or fright are often visible in manifest dream imagery.

The structure of this chapter duplicates the other chapters in its division between theory and practice. Conscious reflections and representations of movement in dreams constitute the content for Section A. These reflections borrow from Symbolist art and literature whilst continuing to draw from Freudian, Jungian and post-Jungian thinking. For the sake of clarity, the theoretical section addresses general and combined movement first, thereafter focusing upon specific movement types in dreams. Consequently, swimming, flying, running and climbing provide headings for the discussion and assist in the preparation for practical application in Section B. Section B begins with an example of a movement dream from a dream journal. After the example, exercises are set that first may assist in coping with fright and flight anxiety responses, and second provide an overall picture of the journey of the psyche through life. The second exercise is adapted and referenced from Joseph Campbell's (2014) *Hero's Journey.*

Section A: Theory: conscious reflections of free and frozen movement

Combined psychic movement

The body operates differently in dreams compared to everyday life. This is because the brain's motor system is alert during wakefulness and relatively subdued in sleep. However, when the unconscious manifests anxiety and presents with sleep walking (which I do not deal with in this book) there is 'reduced inhibitory control' and altered arousal responses (Stallman et al. 2018, p. 106). What I am interested in pursuing here is the *sensation* of movement in a dream and but *not* actually moving. With such sensations the psyche enters a dream space and moves or remains still in different ways. These may combine walking, with running, climbing and swimming or flying; however, I have not yet encountered a dream narrative that combines all of these in one dream or one night of dream sequences. Usually dream narratives that involve movement depend upon the element and space the dream body is in; for example, on low or high ground, inside or outside, in water or in the air. All these elements are also the focus of sensory responses that are dealt with in more detail in Chapter 6.

We have already looked at the places and spaces our psychic selves find themselves in but how they arrived or tried to leave is equally important. Moving with our bodies is a movement through space that involves time; in this way movement forwards, backwards or in circles is a pathway through the spaces of our life experience. Those experiences can be encapsulated in dreams that involve many different types of movement depending on the elements and challenges.

The writings of Nietzsche are a wonderful source of esoteric writing about moving in and through the mythical and metaphoric spaces of life. The ancient Persian religious leader Zarathustra (or Zoroaster) serves as the voice of Nietzsche and speaks his thoughts. As such he writes of coming down from the mountain, along the streams to the sea (Nietzsche 1976). This journey is filled with narrations connecting the earth and its waters with the plight of 'man'kind.[1] Nietzsche's writing has the symbolism of an epic dream, a hero's journey (Campbell 2014). The hero's journey is the symbolic passage of life through all of its obstacles, which will be the basis for an exercise in Section B of this chapter. Below Nietzsche introduces us to the overman.

> Behold, I teach you the overman. The overman is the meaning of the earth. . . . Once the sin against God was the greatest sin; but God died, and these sinners died with him. To sin against the earth is now the most

> dreadful thing, ... Verily, a polluted stream is man. One must be a sea to be able to receive a polluted stream without becoming unclean. Behold, I teach you the overman: he is this sea.
>
> *(Nietzsche 1976, p. 125)*

In the passage quoted above, Nietzsche's infamous statement of God can be seen in context; and it is really the death of belief and the aching loss of faith in something spiritual that is significant here. It may be that civilisation's dismissal of faith in a greater understanding beyond this world brings with it interminable grieving. For dreaming, healing and imaginative arts practice, Nietzsche's poetic writing on the struggle of 'man' and 'overman' is relevant on a metaphysical level. Man can also be understood as the ego (*das Ich*) and overman as the super ego (*das Über Ich*). The struggle through high, low, firm and soft ground is the battle of the self. It is the flight of the soul and its body to move towards individuation. The impediments along the way take on all the elements. The difference between the mountains and valleys with the rivers and sea are binaries that Nietzsche tries to avoid but it is on the mountain where he feels safest yet he also knows that to discover himself truly he needs to come down and enter the waters. Feminist psychoanalyst Luce Irigaray (1991) enters into a conversation with Nietzsche about water, naming his fear and his need for bridges over the water. In this sense the problematic notions of women as fluid and men as solid are called into question. Water as the element for the dreaming body to swim and float in is what I now turn to.

Swimming

Water dreams are doubly uncanny because, in life, water is not the natural element for humans to inhabit; it is the home of water life with its reeds, reefs, rocks and caves. Nonetheless, our conscious bodies are often immersed in water and take pleasure in its coolness on a hot day. The rolling and crashing waves of the ocean also offer wonderful enjoyment to many. But there are times when we are caught in rips or tumbled by a violent wave and we lose the strength to stay afloat. It may be that we are diving and swimming under water and run out of oxygen or that we become too tired and sink. Whatever the conscious experience there will be times when we recall what it is like to be beneath the water's surface, to open our eyes and look out with fear, or with wonder.

When I was a young mother with two very small children, I had recurring dreams of swimming alone deep beneath the surface of dark water making my way through swaying reeds searching for my lost child (see Plate 12 in the colour-plate section at the back of the book). This may have been as a result of my in-laws' farm which had a winding river through rock crevices that were filled with reeds and slippery banks; additionally they bred crocodiles in dams elsewhere on the farm. The dreams continued long after the farm was sold and to this day I am afraid of still dark water. However, the sensation of swimming with a purpose is useful when analysing water dreams. The water of this dream was dense and thick. I could only advance slowly and had to keep moving reeds out of the way. At times I got caught in a strange current and was upside down, at other times I could see faint lights; but I always awoke without finding my child.

In *Water and Dreams*, Bachelard (1983) writes of the 'Charon complex' where death and water combine through the Ancient Greek mythology of the ferryman taking lost souls across the river Styx to Hades. Then there is the related 'Ophelia complex' which develops from the chillingly beautiful image of the drowned Ophelia (from Shakespeare's *Hamlet*) lying in a stream strewn with flowers; Ophelia, Hamlet's love, gives herself back to water and is painted as a floating image of sublime death by the Pre-Raphaelite artist John Everett Millais in 1852. To this end Bachelard (1983) enlarges upon death and water in relation to the poet Rainer Maria Rilke, writing that 'Death in calm water has maternal features' combining water with 'ambivalent images of birth and death' (1983, p. 89). The maternality of water as thick water, blood and maternal milk is also dealt with by Freud (2010, pp. 410, 411) in his explanation of birth dreams and uterine fluids. Freud notes that a child is born out of and into water. From this we can take dreams about immersion in water as signifiers of entering and leaving the world and from a Freudian perspective there is also a longing to return to uterine waters as a place of safety. In this way deep water has strong metaphoric connections with unfathomable pasts and futures. Bachelard (1983, p. 52) writes, 'The past life of the soul is itself a deep water'.

Depth and surface in water can be likened to the unconscious and preconscious. Freud and Jung frequently allude to struggles with interiors and exteriors; in simple terms, an interior could be below the surface, and an exterior above the surface. Jung (2002, p. 194) writes that seeking the hidden treasures of the self is like diving below water. These sought-after treasures or knowledges are always already a part of ourselves and, according to Elizabeth Grosz, it is not so much a returning or a 'reimmersion' but rather a process of actualisation that is required (Bell 2017, p. 3).

The artist Bridgette Minuzzo spends time swimming under water where gravity melts and the body is pulled and pushed with the current. Her images include slow motion videos looking up and through the surface of the water (see Plate 13 in the colour-plate section). 'Vision blurred, hearing muffled, the aquatic realm brings to the fore other senses: balance, spatial awareness, stretch receptors, temperature' (Minuzzo 2017). Bachelard (1983, p. 20) claims that water can contribute to the dual investigation of psychoanalytically 'seeing and revealing oneself'. Water permits imaginative and dynamic intervention compared with the static surface of a mirror; water has movement, light and life which it offers to augment a revelation of the self. 'One cannot dream profoundly with *objects*. To dream profoundly, one must dream with *substances*' (Bachelard 1983, p. 22).[2] Water is a substance and its quality and composition are as important as our movement in, through, with or against it.

When recalling swimming and water dreams, one therefore needs to consider where and how one is moving in the water: underwater, above the water, diving down, coming up, alone, or with another person/object? Other things to consider are the quality and depth of the water; is the water dark, murky, filled with seaweed or river reeds, crystal clear, shallow or deep, cold or tepid? Additionally is it an inland river, a river mouth, the ocean, a swimming pool, the beach, a lake or dam? All of these elements can contribute to capturing the imagery and sensuality of the water and your body moving through it. Then you can ask yourself whether you are breathing freely or not, and have you an oxygen canister as a diver would? Air and water often work together in dreams, and I now turn to the air that is above the water and above the ground as another substance for the sleeping self to move in.

Flying

Flying dreams are my favourite type of dream but this might not be the case for everyone. Freud (1997, p. 256) notes that flying and hovering dreams are usually 'pleasurably toned'. He refers to examples of his patients' dreams where in one instance a woman of shortish stature often dreamed of flying and this was her wish fulfilment for gaining height; another is that of becoming like an angel because the patient had never been called an angel as a child, which was her wish.

Flying can also be associated with freedom. There is that frequent saying, 'free as a bird'. The need to be free is certainly a wish that most people can identify with at times; free from pressures and free from the built environment are examples. Freedom is a subject that will be explored further in the exercises in Section B of this chapter, but the symbolic representations of flying first need to be explored further in this section. For example, the bird or even just its wings are a symbol of flight in many artworks and myths. In Ancient Egyptian mythology, a particular interest of Freud's, the *ba* and the *akh* (sometimes written as *ka*), are two parts of the soul. The *ba* is often represented as half human and half bird hovering above a sarcophagus – the *ba* is capable of flight. In earthly life the *ba* is the guiding conscience and the *aka* is the physical body; in after life the flight of the *ba* takes the deceased further along her/his spiritual journey (Smart 1989). These aspects of flight and rising above the earth are also linked to the cult of the sun and its divine rays. All this is made clear in the famous Egyptian *Book of the Dead* or, more correctly, *The Book of Going Forth by Day* (Smart 1989, p. 199), which is more aptly linked to our discussion on nocturnal dreams that can be revived in the day.

The flight of the soul towards actualisation is another related theme and is used in transpersonal psychology. This is a psychic journey where the spirit and emotions travel, grow and transform into a fully realised all-of-life understanding. Music, dance and poetry are art forms that can assist this soul journey. Soul music, for example, has a deep resonance with trance and transporting oneself to another realm; this type of transportation crosses cultures. For example, instruments from African drums or marimbas to Tibetan singing bowls have sounds that rise from earth to sky enabling the flight of the soul.

Flying needs to be distinguished from falling in dreams. With flying there is a wonderful kind of empowerment, but in falling this power over gravity is lost. 'Dreams of falling are more frequently characterised by anxiety' (Freud 1997, p. 257) and Freud reminds us that 'anxiety in dreams is an anxiety problem and not a dream-problem' (1997, p. 419). As is usually the case with Freud, he looks back to childhood for causes and explains that falling dreams are often associated with the need to be comforted because this is what may have happened when one fell and hurt oneself as a child (1997, p. 257).

There might be also be childhood places that we long for and in our dreams we fly there. The Symbolist artist Marc Chagall left his Russian country village Vitebsk and his flying dreamscapes recall his childhood village experience. This longing is evident in many of Chagall's images, and the spatial arrangement becomes a part of his signature style. This arrangement is one that does not incorporate traditional perspective and laws of gravity. *Blue Circus* (Plate 14 in the colour-plate section) recalls a theatre director and personality in London, Velona Pilcher – a person whom Chagall admired because he loved the theatre, the circus and its magic. The space of *Blue Circus* is beyond the upper realms of the circus tent extending into the deep blue of a night sky. Ultramarine blue provides a space for the jewelled colours of the green horse, yellow moon and crimson trapeze artist. This is a mysterious space of gentle happiness, a space of dreaming and inverted realities.

Running

In a dream one might be running across a desolate landscape, in the middle of traffic, away from a pursuer, or towards an unknown and never reached destination. As with flying and swimming, running in a dream is about the sensations of movement, the feeling of moving ones legs and perhaps also one's arms rapidly through space. In the Introduction to this book, I presented a dream narrative and illustrations from a running dream of my own. In that dream I interrupted, then resumed the running. It seemed as if the manifest content was more about the social interactions than the movement, but when more dream analysis occurs, the running movement lifts the latent content to the fore. The dream then becomes less about running as a fitness activity and more about fleeting time and deadlines. I recall a hollow loneliness in the dream; it was full of people but also seemed filled with silent echoes. Giorgio de Chirico's (1914) surreal dreamscape with a running figure, *The Mystery and Melancholy of the Street*, referred to in Chapter 3, holds a similar kind of vast loneliness where the echoes are as long as the shadows.

Representations of running figures in the history of art quite often also signify heightened emotion or even rebellion. Eugène Delacroix's oil painting *Liberty Leading the People* (1830) is an example of the rising tide of revolution in France. The heroic female figure symbolising liberty flying the French flag and grasping a long bayonet runs over bloodless bodies followed by weapon-wielding followers against the smoking background of Paris. Similarly Pablo Picasso's 1922 painting of two women running, *Two Women Running on the Beach (Race)*, has a statuesque quality; a sense of flight that is simultaneously elated and afraid, two emotions that are often side by side. The monumentality of Picasso's women combined with a vivid movement in space creates the tension of difficult movement in a dream where heaviness and weightlessness conjoin, 'oscillating between two poles: the depiction of the real world and the attempt to look beneath the surface' (Walther 1986, p. 53). Paintings such as these are symbolic of grand movements and changes, just as images captured in dreams can symbolise important or challenging changes in one's life.

Dreams of running on the spot or not being able to move are quite common. Freud (1997, p. 218) writes that the 'sensation of inhibited movement' in dreams is 'closely allied to anxiety'. He also refers to these dream sensations as 'motor paralysis in sleep' (1997, p. 218) which include the inability to move other parts of the body besides the legs. According to Freud (1997, p. 219) such frozen states reflect a 'conflict of will', a kind of refusal or contradiction of what is being asked or expected in the dream. Because one is presumably already lying in a bed, inhibited movement is well suited to the dream where certainty is in abeyance. However, to take Freud's point on anxiety further, the feeling of being frozen in fright, unable to fight back or escape, is an effort of the unconscious to impact upon the preconscious to the significance of existing anxiety. This anxiety is then either supressed or is rendered strong enough to be recalled by the preconscious upon waking.

Climbing

Climbing dreams can sometimes be integrated into running sensations, espe-cially in an escape narrative. They are often related to architecture or the built environment with stairs. The steps might be spiral, interrupted, ladder-like or become like stones set into a cliff, or even down into a cave. In this way climbing can be up or down as a method of seeking something. Therefore, in sync with the rest of this book, the space of the climb can be above or below 'ground'. Her-aclitus, a pre-Socratic Greek philosopher, has a holistic approach to the apparent clash of opposing directions. Hillman cites Heraclitus as follows: "'If you go far enough with any one movement, a countermovement will set in" [and] "The way up and the way down are one and the same"' (Hillman 1979, p. 76). Hillman (1979) reminds us that there are really only two different positions for us: life and death, and even these are not truly opposite (1979, p. 79). Hillman notes that the 'original harmony' between the life drive 'Eros' and the death drive 'Thana-tos' can be restored to an 'ideal balance' through untangling dream fantasies (Hillman 1979, p. 78). With this view, climbing dreams could also be digging dreams, an archaeological activity that is the 'crucial metaphor of psychoanalysis' (Burke 2006, p. 132).

The following discussion on climbing in dreams is therefore as much about space and place, the topic of the previous chapter, as it is about movement. Vidler (1992) writes of certain stairs as a 'vertical labyrinth' (1992, p. 37) and draws on Romanticist and Symbolist writers such as Ernst Theodor Amadeus Hoffman, Arthur Rimbaud, Charles Nodier, Thomas De Quincey and Edgar Allan Poe to illustrate impediments to the desire of rising and reaching up and out from our house of hallucinations. Of these I provide one example I have personally sourced from Hoffman's *The Serapion Brethren* (1908), which shows us an ambivalently poignant and powerful figure noticed by the clerk of the 'Privy Chancery' one 'autumnal' night just before the church clocks struck eleven. The figure stands mournful but proud beneath the 'Townhouse Tower', looking up as if to climb its edifice because there is no answer to his incessantly loud knocking on the door below. The clerk approaches and tells him of his futile attempt because only rats, mice and owls live in the tower. The strange figure wrapped appropriately in black solemnly says he is there to see his beloved. At the first stroke of eleven his beloved appears at the window of the tower high above, and between the first and last chime of the church bells, the stranger accomplishes his psychic reach to make contact with his departed lover. He did not need to enter the tower or climb the stairs.

Vidler (1992) also cites a famous passage on stairs, from De Quincey's *Confessions of an English Opium Eater* where there is a vivid description of Italian engraver Giovanni Battista Piranesi's prison. Words and phrases related to stair dreams are worth requoting from this passage. These include: 'creeping'; 'groping'; 'abrupt termination'; 'a second flight of stairs still higher'; 'and a still more aerial flight of stairs'; 'standing on the brink of the abyss' (De Quincey, in Vidler 1992, p. 37). Piranesi's engravings are terrifyingly complex and include doomed stairways never leading to freedom.

Through a variety of source material including the poets mentioned above and also Freud, Vidler (1992) emphasises the frustration of not being able to climb the stairs or get to the top because 'nothing is finished, nothing is complete or clear' (1992, p. 39). In this way stairs represent an impossible destiny. The stairs might also rise from a dark 'abyssal space' (Vidler 1992, p. 39) so one can be caught on the stairs not being able to go up or down. Freud (1922) writes 'every psycho-physical movement rising above the threshold of consciousness is charged with pleasure . . . and with pain' (1922, p. 3). The pull and push of life and death drives (Eros and Thanatos) are intense in a dream of steep stairways. Freud enlarges on the movement of each of these drives, saying that we rise or descend towards pleasure or pain depending on the limits and thresholds that either of these drives has for us. For example, if our psyche finds pleasure in pain and is drawn to unimaginable risk in order to discover something, this is often referred to as the death drive. Climbing is a metaphor of many things. One is the ill-fated cardinal sin of pride which comes before the Fall. This biblical legend tells of Lucifer, an archangel who wanted equivalence with God and was consequently cast down by fellow archangels to rule the realms of Hell.

In all of the different types of movement and the elements or mediums that occur within, this section has pointed to the tension between oppositional forces and directions. Freud (2010) said that we must always be aware of opposites in dreams; water could be fire, and death could be birth. We are constantly moving between the two. Hillman (1979) contends that we need to work 'through their oppositions' pointing out that oppositions in dreams, and in consciousness are not logical, but neither are they contradictory; they are 'antagonistic and complementary at the same time' (Hillman 1979, p. 75).

With this tension of moving in the push and pull of life's forces, Eros and Thanatos, we continue our movement in Section B. First, there is an example from a dream journal which is followed by exercises on journeys and psychic developments.

Section B: Practical: the unconscious and healing practices – escaping and returning

Escaping and returning is based on survival instincts, with a focus upon retribution and life fulfilment. Below is another example from Joan's dream journal including her accompanying narrative. I also provide a semio-poetic dream analysis of Joan's dream as a basis for the kind of analytical processing you might want to use on your own dream(s). By semio-poetic, I mean an analysis of the line, form, colour, space and texture (these are the 'formal' visual semiotics of an image) in a way that also taps into their poetic and symbolic content. The poetry is in both the visualised and the narrated parts of the dream. It is a method of interpretation that I like to use but you may also want to apply a Jungian interpretation to your dreams devised by Theodor Abt (2005).

Joan's dancing dream

Joan's visual dream journal included the following narrative:

> I have a repetitive dream about tidal/huge waves. The usual scenario is that I'm going about my daily routine when I look over the horizon and see a huge wall of water approaching the shore. The location always varies, sometimes I'm driving up a hill, other times I'm walking along an esplanade.

In the intial dream image (not included here), Joan applied watercolour wash on paper, a sponge was used to blot and repeat the wet paint which is an effective way to work quickly. Compared to the developed image above, the first piece is faint and ephemeral with the blue merging into the white background creating the soft effect of white water. Way below and barely visible are dotted marks in an equally faint orchre with rose hues.

Joan writes:

> According to my subconscious, I forget to nurture myself. I'm constantly trying so damn hard to do things well, to juggle, to achieve, to push through the fatigue of 'trying'. It's too much!! Too much to maintain!! Hence the wave.

The strength of Joan's developed image shows a deliberate attention to self, perhaps a commitment to more self-care and awareness (see Plate 15 in the colour-plate section). It has strong complementary colours in direct contrast to each other, blue and yellow/orange. Whenever colours that are complementary (opposite each other on the colour wheel) are placed side by side, the one intensifies the other. Thus the blue sea and sky is made more vivid by the yellow sand and vice versa. The cool colour of the wave is filled with the power and thunder of its movement, and the heat of the orange yellow provides an opposing force. This sets the scene for the dramatic action of the central figure which Joan sees as dancing. One hand touches a piroetted leg as the other limbs stretch out within an encircling ball of fire light. This tsunami of life is a force encompassing all the elements of sky, water, earth and fire in a survival dance. Eros and Thanatos dance together on the beach in the ever present tension that exists between these two life and death drives.

Interestingly, Joan quotes Nietzsche in her dream narrative: 'I am carried away, my soul dances. Days work! Day's work! Who shall be the lord of the earth?' (Nietzsche 1976, p. 432). This quote comes from the fourth part of *Thus Spoke Zarathustra* where Nietzsche's dialogue with the overman emerges from a dark brooding. In the brooding Nietzsche (1976, p. 432) asks, '*What does the deep midnight delare?*' (italics in the original) and then, as if coming out into the light, he writes what Joan quotes above. However, lingering uncertainty remains with Nietzsche who does not trust the dance on the earth, and calls for flight, 'The moon is cool, the wind is silent. Alas! Alas! Have you flown high enough yet? You have danced: but a leg is no wing' (1976, p. 432). Joan, on the other hand, sees evidence of achievements; she marks the lines which might seem like footprints in the sand but she claims these as dance moves that create 'energy and worthiness'. Perhaps these are 'lines of flight', a Deleuzian movement of freedom and multiplicity? (Deleuze and Guattari 1988). The horizontal arrangement of Joan's composition might testify to a linear journey; however, the circular rim around the figure has its own time, which shares the unbounded movement that Deleuze and Guattari (1988) refer to. This dream and the dreamwork Joan did with it might have helped her subsequent decision to take a leap into the unknown, to travel the world and gain additional experience which required courage. It is a courage that Nietzsche seemed to be trying to harness. Nietzsche, despite his agnosticism, is really calling for a flight of the soul, a release from the world of entrapment and a union with something greater. The movements of the spirit can be combined with the body in an exercise called 'Flight of the Soul' which is outlined in the final exercise of Section B.

Exercises

Your movement dreams

Before embarking on the exercises, you need to go to your own dream journal and find images of movement dreams which you can develop further. Using

Joan's dream image and its accompanying semio-poetic analysis as a guide, here are some questions you can ask of your dream image:

- What type of movement is evident?
- In a running or walking dream you could ask:

  o Is it smooth as a marathon runner runs before fatigue sets in, a calm rhythm without much energy being expended, barely lifting the feet, just floating across the ground?
  o Or can the jarring of joints be felt as the ground is pounded and a stitch grips the core muscles?
  o What type of surface can be felt, if any?
  o Are the feet bare or shod, can the sand, earth, grass, be felt beneath the feet?
  o And again, who is with you, if anyone?

- In a flying dream you could ask:

  o Where is that flight?
  o Is it in the garden, a room, over the city, over the ocean, or somewhere else?
  o Is the flying assisted by someone or something?
  o Is it hovering, floating, or moving swiftly?

- Ask similar and relevant questions of swimming and climbing dreams and also refer to Section A of this chapter for inspiration with your interpretation.
- The space or place of that dream will assist in capturing some of the imagery and give it form.
- The type of movement can suggest the kind of brushstroke, or quality of medium and material chosen for the representation.
- Additionally the method of moving combined with the location can inform the choice of colour and form.

Materials: There are a few options depending on your preferred creative medium of expression (e.g. art, poetry, music, drama, dance).

- An A3 or A4 unlined good-quality visual art journal; pencils, pens, coloured pencils, watercolour or acrylic paints. Glue, scissors and collage materials of your choice.
- A journal for creative writing with illustrations. This could be suitable for a short story, or long poem, a drama script, a song, a dance choreography. For dance *5 Rhythms* is a wonderful resource for personalising your body's movement through space in response to emotions (Juhan 2003).
- A music manuscript book for musical composition and a keyboard or instrument of your choice.

Epic journeys: searching and finding

In this exploration I use Joseph Campbell's well-known *Hero's Journey* as a model (Campbell 2003). It is a typical 'quest' story line, which can also be found in Christopher Booker's *The Seven Basic Plots* (2004). You may also refer to Richard Wagner's operas with their other worldly musical wanders of dramatic love, loss and redemption. In your own hero's journey you are guided to illustrate your life journey (or significant part thereof) symbolically through visually realised spaces that can be a combination of landscapes, townscapes or any part of the earth, skies and seas that might be useful to your journeying.

A few words before you begin: You might not be emotionally ready to do this exercise; it involves deep work that could bring up aspects of your life that you are not fully prepared to revisit. In therapy, the life journey or heroic journey is not a process that is undertaken at the beginning of a therapeutic programme which usually involves several sessions. The therapist and client need to have a firm relationship of trust and this is now the same for you because you're essentially doing therapy on yourself. You need to trust yourself. You also need to have back-up. By that I mean someone you can call or who is there for you as you work through the exercise which might even take you weeks or months to complete, depending on the difficulties encountered on the way. When you feel you are ready, then commit to completing the exercise; you do not need to give yourself a strict time frame, just a promise to complete all the steps honestly with yourself.

The steps:

1   Choose a metaphor for yourself. This will help with your visualisation, illustration and processing. You could choose your favourite animal, or even a plant. Choose something that you are able to imbue with a personality. For example, when I first did this exercise myself, I chose a little star in the night sky. It's important that you give the metaphor the ability to move (walk, run, swim, fly, or all of these). If you like you can name it, but avoid using a human name to prevent accidental associations along the way; maintain the metaphor so that the journey is symbolic. For the purpose of the following instructions I will just use '0'.

2   The ordinary, everyday world:

   •   Depending on whether you want to work from the present or a past stage, you need to ask yourself: What is this ordinary world? What does it look like? Where is 0 in this world? What is 0 surrounded by? What is 0 doing?

   •   In the first page of your journal: draw, paint, collage, compose or write 0 in the ordinary world, paying careful attention to detail. It may help if you speak to 0 and ask 0 the questions above to really understand what is required in this representation of 0's ordinary world at that/this time.

   •   Everything included in the image is a symbol of something beyond itself. For example a tree is not just a tree, it's a symbol of growth, oxygen and rooted living; it holds memories and has witnessed many things if it is a large tree. If it is a young tree, or a dying tree, these aspects mean different things respectively. Take your time, this does not need to be done in one session.

3   The call:

- 0 is challenged to move out of the ordinary world, to go somewhere or to do something necessary, it is usually something that needs to be found and restored to its rightful place. This call might be whispered from the mountains, echo in caves, or rise up like a song from deep within 0's personal well.
- Again, you need to listen. Where is/did the call come from? What is/was the message?
- In the second page of your journal, draw, paint, collage, write or compose a representation of the call in relation to 0. Pay attention to detail as always, and especially to space. How much space is there between 0 and the origin of the call? Keep to symbolic imagery; for example, the call can be a white light or a burning flame, a chiming clock or a bell peal.

4   Reluctance:

- 0 is faced with the unknown and is fearful. 0 may look out and see a vastness or a perilous terrain. 0 is not sure of the route or how long it will take to achieve what is necessary.
- Be still with 0. Now is a good time to do one of the meditation exercises elsewhere in this book. These can be found in the 'Guided Meditation' exercise in Section B of Chapter 3, or the 'States of Consciousness' exercise in Section B of Chapter 1, or the 'Visualisation' process also in Section B of Chapter 1. Be kind to yourself and to 0. Breathe mindfully throughout this exercise.
- When you are ready, turn to the third page of your journal and draw, paint, compose or write about 0 in this stage of refusal. It is a psychic paralysis because of what 0 sees ahead. Represent 0 in the vastness, the depths, the road into the distance, or whatever it is that 0 is looking into. In essence you will be representing fear and the unknown, so it might be quite abstract.

5   Meeting your mentor:

- Help comes to 0 out of the vastness of the unknown. This is someone or something that needs to be represented in your journal so consider what this form of wisdom might look like. You might want to use one of your archetypes from Chapter 2; you may prefer to maintain an abstract and symbolic theme that you have already begun in 'ordinary world' representation.

- When you are as certain as you can be of what 0's wise voice looks like, go to the fourth page of your journal and draw, paint, collage, compose or write your mentor into the road or journey that lies ahead.
- Whilst you are in the process of representing the mentor in your journal, pay attention to feelings, your body and your breath. 0's strength has been identified and this is a time to feel the power of real courage and commitment to the task and journey ahead.

6   Crossing the threshold:

- The previously unknown starts to take shape for 0 as 0 ventures forth. It is nothing like the ordinary world. It has forms, colours, lines, shadows, textures and perspectives that are new, some of which are threatening. Spend some time considering what 0 sees and whether 0 is listening to the mentor. Has the mentor left?
- Again, being mindful of how you feel and taking time to be gentle with yourself, take courage as you now move to page five of your journal, the first page of the difficult journey and experiences which 0 is now aware of. This is what you need to represent on the page, with drawing, painting, collage, poetry or music. In musical composition there needs to be a distinct shift in the colour, tone and tempo. There could be a sense of real movement in this representation, so consider the terrain carefully. Remember that giving form to something is a way of naming it, recognising it and dealing with it, so take pride in the courage 0 has.

7   Tests, allies and enemies:

- This is when things start to happen and 0 is confronted with ordeals. At times 0 is not clear who is a friend or who is a foe. It is confusing and there are many symbolic hoops to jump through. Spend time considering what needs to be included. Again you will be giving form to aspects of 0's journey that might have been long buried or forgotten so be brave and take your time.
- You are now on page six of your journal and it might seem that you need a couple of pages for this stage, a double spread perhaps. If your medium is music, this might be to quicken the tempo and include more dynamic contrasts. Consider encapsulating all the trials and confusions into one page; for example, it could be a useful exercise to group things but it also might be more useful to distinguish the separate 'enemies' and the separate friends. Is it necessary to re-introduce the mentor? What do the tests look like? Are there crossroads, bridges, boats? These can be dealt with as symbolically as it suits.
- There will be moments of weakness and moments of strength in this for 0. Try to represent each with respect and truth to 0.

8 The approach:

- 0 is close to what is often called the 'inmost cave' in the heroic journey. This cave symbolises what encloses the secret or the key to the challenge. It also encloses 0's greatest fear but that is not yet clear. What does the situation look like now that 0 is almost there? Try to visualise how the covering of secrecy might be represented.
- Turn to a clean page in your journal following the 'tests, allies and enemies' representation, and draw, paint, collage, compose musically or poetically the approach to the cave. Remember to consult with 0 so that the emotions of that approach are captured in front of the cave. Is 0 alone again?
- Be mindful of your own feelings. Are there fight and flight triggers? Take care to be gentle with yourself. Take this as slowly as you need to so that you are prepared for the next stage.

9 The ordeal:

- Fear in its raw form is exposed. 0 experiences and confronts it. What is this fear? Why did it lie hidden so far away? What does this secret fear look like? Is there anything good in this cave? Look for a light or something that is lit with kindness and not menace. How can 0 reach that? What is in the way?
- Be still with 0. Be still with yourself. Find a rhythm in your breathing, feeling the good clean spirit of courage and kindness fill your lungs, veins and body, and the clotted, old, bad air leave and go out the window.
- When you are ready, go to the page in your journal where you can relate and represent this ordeal. Give form, colour, line, depth, texture and sound to what is in this cave and what happens in the cave. This is a moment in most art forms where there is a crescendo; it is both the highest and the lowest point.

10 The reward:

- 0 has grasped the symbolic treasure that had to be fought for. Much was endured to reach this point. It is a moment that 0 might want to last and so you may want to prolong this moment in your representation.
- Reach for your journal and celebrate this climax for 0. With your choice of medium, create the moment of triumph. In an orchestra, this is usually when one hears more of the brass instruments. However, you might prefer it to be a quiet moment when there is time to pause. Whatever your choice of colour, line, form, texture or volume, represent this as 0 felt it at that time.

11 The return:

- It is not over yet. 0 has to get back and danger lurks on the road back. 0 has the reward but there are forces that want to take it away and/or prevent the safe return.

- What does the return journey look like in symbolic form? Try to visu-alise and feel what 0 saw, heard and felt on the brink of return with the precious reward. Consider how you want to show 0 both commencing and enduring the return. What is met on the way? How is it dealt with? Are there temptations? What do all of these look like?
- In the next free page of your journal, you can now draw, paint, collage, compose poetically or musically this return journey. Consider whether 0 is exhausted or injured; it's likely there will be some wounds. What form do you want to give them?
- Be aware that after a trauma there are scars and they do not go away quickly, they need to be cared for. Perhaps 0 requires help, which arrives in symbolic forms. What are these symbols? Represent this important road to recovery as clearly as you can, it will have many reference points for 0 to be restored and find the strength to return home with the treasure.

12 Emergency and emergence:

- This is another threshold for 0 who is nearly home but faces an ordeal, perhaps a breakdown which is a severe trial to 0's strength. It is tough after all 0 has been through, still carrying the reward but not knowing how to use it.
- 0 is once again in crisis. What does this look, sound and feel like? Tap into the symbols that might be visible. There is first an emergency, a panic not to lose what is found, and then an emergence once the ordeal is over. 0 survives.
- In the next free page of your journal, represent 0 at this moment of cri-sis and survival in line, colour, form and texture, in drawing, painting, collage, poetry, prose or music. For more information on psychic or spiritual emergency and emergence (as opposed to psychosis) refer to the work of Grof and Grof (1985, 1991).

13 The ordinary world with new power:

- 0 is back home. After arriving, there is another transformation as 0 learns how to use the treasure that was so difficult to find and bring back safely. If 0 does not use the new power appropriately it will fail and have dif-ficult consequences so that 0 may need to repeat the whole journey again. That should be guarded against, as often there is an unnecessary cycle. However, if it's necessary for real healing to take place, the journey can be repeated and 0 will return even stronger. Either way if the treasure is trea-sured and used well, 0 can share knowledge of the wonder 0 knows exists outside of the ordinary world and live a more fulfilled life as a result.

Flight of the soul [3]

This exercise extends Erik Erikson's developmental stages of life so that the journey is more cyclic and continuous than linear and you are able to conceive of birth, life and death as a rhythm of existence in what might be a wider realm. Erikson's stages are useful to list here as a reference and/or comparison: (1) Infancy (trust versus mistrust); (2) Early Childhood (autonomy versus shame and doubt); (3) Play Age (initiative versus guilt); (4) School Age (industry versus inferiority); (5) Adolescence (identity and repudiation versus identity diffusion); (6) Young Adult (intimacy and solidarity versus isolation); (7) Adult (generativity versus self-absorption); (8) Mature Age (integrity versus despair) (Erikson 1980).

When I first tried it I made a few pencil drawings of how I imagine the before, during and aftermath of my life. They are illustrated below as examples. Later I used clay to augment some of the phases which I also include as examples. Crucial stages should include times when your body and soul grow. This exercise delves into your childhood and if there are aspects of those times that are troubling, or perhaps a mystery, then you should ensure that you have emotional support when you undertake this exercise. The creative process can lift hidden aspects and you need to be ready for what additional self-care may be required. Although it's called flight of the soul, the body must not be neglected so it's necessary to be aware of lightness and heaviness when the life stages shift, take flight or linger.

Art materials: Art and creative materials are the same as those provided earlier in this section. However, 'flight of the soul' is also a lifespan exercise. This is why you may want to work in three dimensions. Some suggestions include:

- Clay or a modelling medium which works well with the fluidity of 'flight of the soul'.
- Carving a series of avocado pear stones. Simple wood or lino cutting tools are fine.
- Creating a staged life scene in a tub of sea or river sand. A few small objects that can metaphorically symbolise you and your life's stages are required.

Process and documentation:

- Take a photograph of each stage; this is especially important for the sand tray so you have a record before you move to the next stage. When smoothing the sand over for the next stage, do so mindfully so that it's not an abrupt erasure.
- Sometimes, it's perfect just to stay with the moment in the sand tray; with its dips and mounds, what is buried and what stands out; all will speak to you of particular times in your life's journey.
- Always ask yourself, how was my body then and where was my soul?
- You can then assemble or collage the images and process them as you feel you need to, always acknowledging how far you have come.

Examples of the stages:

Stage 1: Pre-birth and Birth. This visualising a time beyond memory is like dreaming, and needs to actively tap into the unconscious using a technique that works – a

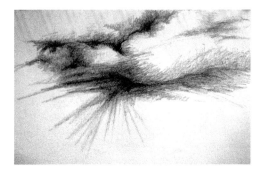

FIGURE 4.1 Kathleen Connellan (2014), *Stage 1 of Flight of the Soul: Pre-birth and Birth*, graphite pencil in an art journal.

Author's own artwork.

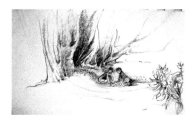

FIGURE 4.2 Kathleen Connellan (2014), *Stage 2 of Flight of the Soul: Childhood*, graphite pencil in an art journal.

Author's own artwork.

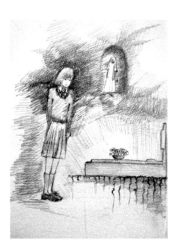

FIGURE 4.3 Connellan, Kathleen (2014), *Stage 3 of Flight of the Soul: Initiation*, graphite pencil in an art journal.

Author's own artwork.

meditation exercise could help. For me the place of my soul with its unborn body is in a free space with both light and clouds.

Stage 2: Childhood. This is literal memory of my childhood with some symbolic content. As pre-school children my brother and I used to play intently together beneath large trees. My soul is very much in the garden in these early years; beyond the trees are many flowers that provided a fantasy world.

Stage 3: Initiation. The stage of initiation into the world of reality, when the soul experiences sorrow and pain and the fantasy of flowers seems distant,

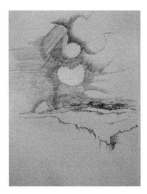

FIGURE 4.4 Kathleen Connellan (2014), *Stage 4 of Flight of the Soul: Adolescence*, graphite pencil in an art journal.

Author's own artwork.

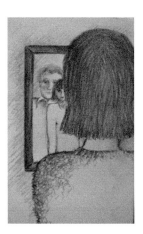

FIGURE 4.5 Kathleen Connellan (2014), *Stage 5 of Flight of the Soul: Adulthood 1*, graphite pencil in an art journal.

Author's own artwork.

is visualised here. I represent myself at convent boarding school grieving for my older sister who was killed tragically. This is a time when my soul hovered and the body felt heavy.

Stage 4: Adolescence. Adolescence is a significant soul and body shift. My visualisation of this period presents a dominant sky in a landscape that seems to have distant and dark mountains as a destiny.

Stage 5: Adulthood 1. The first stage of adulthood seems to be literally portrayed here. This stage is sometimes referred to as that of 'union' because it is when a soul mate might be found and a long life relationship may ensue.

Stage 6: Adulthood 2. The second stage of adulthood is shown here as if the mountains are close, but the presence of a single street lamp provides an ambiguous and symbolic presence. Drawing symbolically helps to situate the soul. The lamp could symbolise the eye of modernity in a landscape of potential.

Stage 7: Death. Death is portrayed here as a time when the soul is both of the earth, the sky and the sea. Again it is the symbolism of the landscape that gives the soul space for flight.

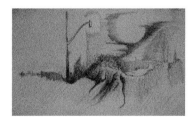

FIGURE 4.6 Kathleen Connellan (2014), *Stage 6 of Flight of the Soul: Adulthood 2*, graphite pencil in an art journal.

Author's own artwork.

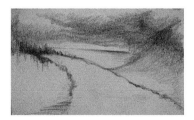

FIGURE 4.7 Connellan, Kathleen (2014), *Stage 7 of Flight of the Soul: Death,* graphite pencil in an art journal.

Author's own artwork.

Figures 4.8–4.11 show clay examples of some stages in the above exercise.

Clay is useful if you want to concentrate on a more obvious unity of body and soul, particularly for parenthood stages in adulthood. The stages portrayed here are those of trying to be a mother and care for a family. In one stage I wanted the clay figure to stand up but she symbolically collapsed so it felt right to bring her down into a more solid seated position. The clay was never fired but rather returned ceremonially to the earth.

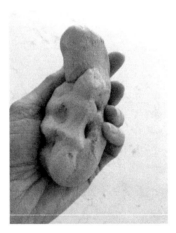

FIGURE 4.8 Kathleen Connellan (2014), *Stage 1 of Flight of the Soul: pre-birth and birth*, unfired clay.

Author's own artwork.

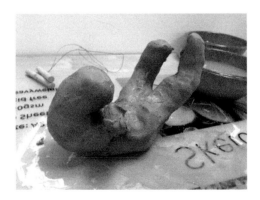

FIGURE 4.9 Kathleen Connellan (2014), *Stage 2 of Flight of the Soul: Childhood*, unfired clay.

Author's own artwork.

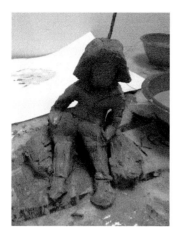

FIGURE 4.10 Kathleen Connellan (2014), *Stage 3 of Flight of the Soul: Adulthood 1*, unfired clay.

Author's own artwork.

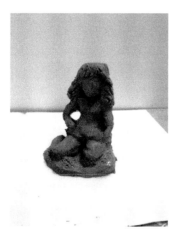

FIGURE 4.11 Kathleen Connellan (2014), *Stage 4 of Flight of the Soul: Adulthood 2*, unfired clay.

Author's own artwork.

Conclusion

This chapter has taken us swimming, flying, running, climbing or fixed to one spot. Movement in dreams is the psychic movement of the self through experience. It is as much about movement as it is about non-movement and consequently is often a struggle. The sensation of moving without movement is a powerful trope in such dreams which blend the strange obsessions brought to the psyche through sleep. There are alternate triumphs and fears of rising or sinking and the terrors of frozen movement. Above all there is the 'impassable network of broken connections' (Vidler 1992, p. 40) and the primal need to return to a place of safety. The psyche uses the elements of water and air as mediums to swim or fly in search of security and liberation. It is the liberating quality that is so important for creative practice. Creatively working with dreams of movement provides opportunities to rise out of the constraining instincts within the unconscious. Many examples were provided in Sections A and B to offer inspiration for creative avenues. The exercises should help you retrace your steps symbolically through life to recover what might have been lost or recognise what needs to be left behind and what needs to be embraced. Turning the explorations into artworks can be a culmination and celebration of who you are.

Notes

1 The gendered 'man' could be interpreted neutrally by readers and typical of nineteenth-century writing but it's worth considering feminist readings of such generalisations through Luce Irigaray (1991).
2 One cannot dream solely with objects, one also has to engage with the matter, substance, the material and the immaterial. The object in dreams is the topic of Chapter 5.
3 'Flight of the soul' is not my own phrase; it comes from a Shamanic paradigm that I do not specifically engage with in the chapter. However, ancient traditions of trance and trance-dance can be extremely healing and readers can explore their own creativity to arrive at these. There is also a YouTube dance/music video by Stive Morgan called 'Flight of the Soul' from the *New Galactic* album (2012).

References

Abt, T. (2005), *Introduction to Picture Interpretation: According to C.G. Jung*. Living Human Heritage, Zurich.

Bachelard, G. (1983), *Water and Dreams: An essay on the imagination of matter*, trans. E.R. Farrell, Pegasus, Dallas.

Bell, V. (2017), 'An interview with Elizabeth Grosz: "the incorporeal"', *Theory, Culture & Society*, vol. 34, no. 7–8, pp. 237–243.

Booker, C. (2004), *The Seven Basic Plots: Why we tell stories*, Continuum, London.

Burke, J. (2006), *The Gods of Freud: Sigmund Freud's Art Collection*, Knopf, Sydney.

Campbell, J. (2014), *The Hero's Journey: Joseph Campbell on His Life and Work: The Collected Works of Joseph Campbell*, ed. P. Cousineau, New World Library, Novato.

Cannon, W.B. (1914), 'The interrelations of emotions as suggested by recent physiological researches', *The American Journal of Psychology*, vol. 25, no. 2, pp. 256–282.

Deleuze G. and Guattari, F. (1988), *A Thousand Plateaus: Capitalism and schizophrenia*, trans. B Massumi, Continuum, London.

Erikson, E. (1980), *Identity and the Life Cycle*, Norton, New York.

Freud, S. (1922), *Beyond the Pleasure Principle*, trans. C.J.M. Hubback, The International Psycho-Analytic Press, London, Ovid PsychBooks.

Freud, S. (1997), *The Interpretation of Dreams*, trans. A.A. Brill, Wordsworth Classics, Ware.

Freud, S. (2010), *The Interpretation of Dreams*, trans. J. Strachey, Basic Books, New York.

Grof, S. and Grof, C. (1985), 'Forms of spiritual emergency: the spiritual emergency', *Network Newsletter*, Spring, pp. 1–2.

Grof, S. and Grof, C. (1991), *The Stormy Search for Self: Understanding and living with spiritual emergency*, Mandala, London.

Hillman, J. (1979), *The Dream and the Underworld*, Harper & Row, New York.

Hoffman, E.T.A. (1908), *The Serapion Brethren Vol. 1*, trans. A. Ewing, George Bell & Sons, London, Project Gutenberg eBooks.

Irigaray, L. (1991), *Marine Lover of Friedrich Nietzsche*, trans. G.C. Gill, Columbia University Press, New York.

Juhan, A. (2003), *Open Floor: Dance, therapy, and transformation through the 5rhythms*, Union Institute University, Cincinnati.

Jung, C.G. (2002), *Dreams*, trans. R.F.C. Hull, Routledge, London.

Nietzsche, F. (1976), *The Portable Nietzsche*, trans. W. Kaufmann, Penguin, Harmondsworth.

Minuzzo, B. (2017), *Sound, Water, Waves*, exhibition catalogue, South Australian School of Art Gallery, Adelaide.

Morgan, S. (2012), 'Flight of the Soul', music video, YouTube, viewed 18 July 2018, www.youtube.com/watch?v=ylfQR7k9XQ.

Siegal, D. (2010), *Mindsight: Transform your brain with the science of human kindness*, Oneworld, Oxford.

Smart, N. (1989), *The World's Religions*, Cambridge University Press, Cambridge.

Stallman, H.M., Kohler, M. and White, J. (2018), 'Medication induced sleepwalking: a systematic review', *Sleep Medicine Reviews*, vol. 37, pp. 105–113.

Vidler, A. (1992), *The Architectural Uncanny: Essays in the modern unhomely*, MIT Press, Cambridge.

Walther, I.F. (1986), *Picasso: Genius of the century*, Taschen, Cologne.

5

THE OBJECT AND ITS CRISIS[1]

Locating pain and pleasure

Introduction

This chapter uses some of the theories put forward by the art movement that is central to dream-work and imaginative arts practice, i.e. Surrealism. The unwanted or unsolicited object (*l'object insolité*) is the term used in Surrealism; and in Jungian language it is the 'object-imago' (Jung 2002, p. 62). My aim is to use the object-imago as a bridge between levels of consciousness. The object-imago is a dream object, which carries memories and desires and it can be simultaneously familiar and unfamiliar. What the chapter also addresses are actual objects in the real world such as a vase or sculpture in the home. This tangible object may have been obtained either from the desire to possess it or because it found its place with you and became imbued with memory. The dream object and the object of desire or memory share meaning because they both have significance in your life. Therefore the dream object and the tangible object are dealt with together in this chapter because there are psychic overlaps. The dream object lives in the unconscious and the tangible object presides in the conscious; the dream object needs to be actualised into material reality and brought into the conscious realm to be fully comprehended.

This chapter, like the preceding ones, has both a theoretical and a practical section. Section A, the theoretical section, uses visual examples from contemporary art that could be described as surreal. These include objects in disguise and out of place or proportion. As mentioned, the Surrealist art movement from the twentieth century is the backdrop for the theoretical discussion. Contemporary artist Jasmine Symons' images reveal powers of ambiguity and symbolic communication. Although these images might have been completed in a conscious and waking state of mind, they are very close to Section B's unconscious images and explanations taken directly from dream journals. As a means of situating the object in crisis, the concept of fetish is also a focus. The fetish object is discussed using Freud and Lacan's ideas on lack and desire, where a group of objects or a single object could be symbolic of loss. The art images in Section A show how dreamed and imagined objects transfer and project meaning. Therefore we experience finished works of art in Section A and take a step back in Section B, where the relatively unfinished images of a dream are illustrated.

Section B, the practical section, first provides an example of one illustrated and narrated dream for the reader. The dream script locates and links sites of pleasure and pain. An analysis of the dream then reveals the dream objects as projections of both desire and denial; first in the realm of the known (conscious realities of everyday life and experience), and second in the unknown or lodged in the unconscious. In this way the unsolicited object is recognised as the object of desire, or alternatively the object to be feared. The second part of Section B is devoted to practical exercises; these are designed to be healing practices although some may be initially confronting depending on the content you use. The first exercise is a technique devised by Surrealist artist Salvador Dali called 'the paranoiac critical method', which will be explained in the exercise's instructions. The second exercise is a collaborative one which involves at least two participants to make it worthwhile. It also originates from Surrealism and is called 'the exquisite corpse'; instructions will be provided with the exercise. Additional text accompanies all exercises to help with processes of healing where uncomfortable objects manifest.

Section A: Theory: conscious reflections on the object and its crisis

Sublimation

For the purposes of this chapter the objects in crisis are not represented as obviously human figures or animals but instead as apparently inanimate things. This is to facilitate understanding of the substitution and sublimation that takes place when an object is not what it seems and can (upon further dream analysis) actually represent the dreamer. This unsolicited object is more than just a 'strange object' (see below excerpt), it is the uninvited object that arrives from another context and spatial hierarchy and may seem alien.

> Dreams are by nature conducive to the 'creation' of strange objects; needless to say, the surrealists did not discover this phenomenon, nor were they the first to utilize it. But they are the originators of a new type of relationship between the dream-object and man, in which this object progressively asserts its concrete existence in man's world and, consequently, begins to interfere in an active manner in man's spiritual existence.
>
> *(Finkelstein 1979, p. 20)*

The effects of objects that appear 'out of nowhere' in dreams and mental meanderings can upset one's equilibrium. An object that is not specifically recognisable as a particular person or animal but is perhaps a jug, a rope, a pair of spectacles, a pen, which arrives on a scene and may appear larger than it 'should' or be in quite the 'wrong' place, immediately takes on a significant symbolism in the dream narrative. It becomes a foreground object in that dream space, and is not part of the murky dream background. It demands to be seen and acknowledged. In some ways this demand is only evident after deciphering that the object is in the guise of something else, that it can be two or more objects at once depending on how it is perceived.

This leads us into the representation of such objects in Surrealist and surreal-style painting. The object in these paintings was previously overlooked; it is now recognised despite an apparent disguise. An example can be seen in Plates 16, 17 and 18 in the colour-plate section at the back of the book).

The initial object that inserted a forceful presence to the artist Jasmine Symons is the electric power meter (Plate 16). This solid block of connectivity was an essential fixture, which, because of its position in the home, was the first thing the artist saw when she awoke in the morning. It assumed a character of its own, 'a stalker in a balaclava' (Symons 2016), which became the catalyst for two more paintings (Plates 17 and 18) with additional layers of ambiguity. Initially, the power meter harboured a watchful but ominous anger. It fixed its stare unrelentingly but would not release its disguise. Three years later, and through the process of sublimation the object (Plate 17) assumed a semi-human form (Symons 2016). The artist identifies the form as a troubled mother in the 1940s. The background wallpaper is a fictional haze of domesticity and the white outline creates a hovering effect of uncertainty. The power meter's head, neck and shoulders sit strangely behind the armless, legless body which is a shiny pink corset strapped in a central stance of bondage. One year on (Plate 18) the form reappears more starkly against a crisp wallpaper that seems to assert its domestic trope but this semblance of home is contradicted by the form's unchanged posture of repression.

Surreal forms are often painted in unreal proportion or in an unsettling pictorial space. An example of such pictorial space is the commanding frontality of Symons' versions of *Armless* (Plates 17 and 18). Additionally in twentieth-century Surrealism, René Magritte's 1952 oil painting *The Listening Room* portrays a single green apple filling a room from ceiling to floor and wall to wall. This is the object-imago in a claustrophobic space. It is imagined and then presented as huge because of the space it occupies in the consciousness of the subject. The disjuncture between the object and its space is symptomatic of a world closing in on Magritte and the viewer. Magritte used familiar objects like the apple because people have either forgotten to notice what is in front of them or lost sight of the real object (Finkelman 2010, p. 169). In this way the apple masks reality. Another well-known Surrealist object is a fur covered tea cup and saucer by Meret Oppenheim (1936) simply called *Object*. One's trained sensory response is initially disturbed when forced to reconsider the purpose of an otherwise functional object. Apparently the cup was inspired by a conversation between Picasso and the artist at a Paris café regarding her fur-covered bracelet; she reputedly said that you can cover anything with fur, 'even this cup'. She used the fur of a Chinese gazelle to cover the cup and saucer which she then put into the first Surrealism show dedicated to objects (Caws 2011, p. 25).

Sometimes the objects are not only in disguise or deformed, they are almost unrecognisable and abstracted in art. Lucy Lippard (1997) and many other arts writers have written about the retreat of the object in conceptual and abstract art. In the height of non-representational art from the late twentieth century into the twenty-first century, it became unfashionable for artists to show anything that might be too literal. This representational flight from recognisable reality resulted in decades of experimental conceptual art that became more and more difficult for ordinary people to understand. This did not mean that the object had disappeared from art; it had just been suspended from visible and representative reality. Lippard's (1970) writing on the Surrealists' struggle with what is there and what is not there throws some light on the object that is really an object of need or desire. She writes that the

> object exists outside us, without our taking part in it . . . the object assumes the immovable shape of desire and acts upon our contemplation . . . the object is movable and such that it can be acted upon . . . the object tends to bring about our fusion with it and makes us pursue the formation of a unity with it.
>
> *(Lippard 1970, p. 96)*

When considering the fusion of an object with the self or an(other) self, for example one's mother, it is useful to include Lacan's thinking on sublimation (Lacan 2006). Lacan writes that sublimation 'designates an identificatory reshaping of the subject' (2006, p. 95). In other words, as subjects we can reshape ourselves according to attributes of the found object, also known as *l'objet trouvé* in art. In this way we engage in 'intersubjective' communication between one part of the self and an 'other' (Lacan 2006, p. 30). The actual process of sublimation takes something ordinary, like the power meter in Symons' paintings, into the extraordinary. This extraordinary aspect can be darkly melancholic or reasonably benign, involving past longings and future strivings. For Lacan, the process of sublimation assists in healing and is a release from mental suffering particularly related to loss. The whole process is part of the Lacanian 'symbolic chain' where the real, the symbolic and the imaginary communicate with each other and with the outer world of objects (Lacan 2006).

Inner and outer worlds are symbolically connected through art which can substitute for different types of loss. Levine (2008) says that we might be looking at 'nothing more than a lowly still-life painting of pots and pans but its pictorial refashioning as the material signifier of an absent present might transform the work into an amazing masterpiece' (Levine 2008, p. 32). For example, Hal Foster (1992) claims that seventeenth-century Dutch still-life paintings were commissioned to be painted in a way that substituted a lost religious aura. The Dutch Protestants had rejected the Catholic belief in God's presence on the altar with its shimmering sacramental chalices. The absence of that splendid religious symbolism created a void in their lives which was filled with the mysteriously beautiful still-life paintings that subsequently adorned their domestic spheres. Foster calls this an 'inversion of the subject – object relations . . . as if the objects were endowed with life to the degree that the viewer is sapped of it' (Foster 1992, p. 7).

From the above it can be gleaned that it is not only in making art, and thereby transcending ordinary reality in the creative process, but also when one is in the presence of such art objects that sublimation can occur. 'One of the unexpectedly important things that art can do for us is to teach us how to suffer more successfully' (de Botton and Armstrong 2013, p. 26). To see our sadness in a simple domestic painting or in an abstracted sculpture that speaks of universal tragedy is to invite a process of healing sublimation. Nonetheless, the therapeutic benefits of sublimation can only take full effect if we have first done the necessary work to know ourselves as discussed in Chapters 1and 2 of this book.

Fetish

Fetishism is when sublimation is consciously willed. Fetishism and sublimation are therefore connected but it will help to look at the fetish-as-object separately and then return to how the two are related.

As stated above, the fetish is not necessarily the unsolicited object but rather the solicited object; it is an object that is sought as a replacement for something that may or may not be known. For Freud, the ego and the object can prove inseparable especially if the object is attached to suffering (Freud 1963, p. 4). For example, according to Freud (1927), if the absent thing is not acknowledged or dealt with, this is a disavowal, '*Verluegnung*' (Freud 1927, p. 150). In such instances the subject takes no responsibility for the loss or absence which can also be displaced, '*Verdrängung*' (Freud 1927, p. 153). However, whether the missing object is disavowed or displaced, it is still felt; its affect remains and that is why the fetish is sought.

The etymological origins of the term fetish derive from the Latin *facticius*, as well as the French and Middle English *fetis*, which is something that is elegantly and handsomely made. Its meaning also relates to making something artificial; this can be broken down to art – artifice – artificial. However, according to the online etymological dictionary and also the *Webster's Dictionary* from 1880, the specific term came to English via Portuguese traders and sailors returning from the Guinea coast of Africa with knowledge of charms and talismans; these *feitiço* could be material objects including those in nature such as stones, trees, and even an animal alive or dead. In this sense an 'object' that becomes a fetish has more to it than its materiality; it holds a symbolism that is believed to carry spiritual powers for many purposes. It is this anthropological understanding of fetish that I use here in Chapter 5.[2]

The power-carrying object is also the object-imago which is not dissimilar to the archetype discussed in Chapter 2. However, as stated earlier, the focus here is on an inanimate object. That object can become fixated upon without the subject (the person) really understanding why it is essential to possess the object. Jung (2002) notes that if the object were removed the psychological effects would be extreme. However, he adds: 'The subject's unconscious projections, which canalized unconscious contents into the imago and identified it with the object, outlive the actual loss of the object' (Jung 2002, p. 62). In other words powerful spiritual forces are active in our unconscious and are partially projected out and directed into suitable container objects in the conscious; nonetheless a residue always remains within the person's unconscious.

It is arguable that Freud's extensive personal collection of art objects were fetish objects. He collected obsessively and even took some of his statuettes on holiday with him (Burke 2006, p. 301). Freud's acquisitions were predominantly archaeo-logical finds from Ancient Egypt and Greece, and they often had missing limbs. Although the missing parts resulted from damage over the centuries, the usually small statues hold a tense blend of power and loss. For example, his small Roman bronze copy of Athena is 'pitted and scored' and this goddess of war is missing her spear (Burke 2006, p. 92). The absent spear in the context of Freud's work on loss is more powerful than a present spear. Freud's art collection is predominantly made up of figurines acquired in the late nineteenth century when the finds from ancient tombs were being sold relatively cheaply. Freud was more than a collector; there was an urgency in his need to populate his consulting room with past gods. He used them constantly in therapy, picking them up and offering them to his patients to hold (Burke 2006, p. 312). They were silent speaking objects that harboured millennial myths and mysteries that he wanted his patients to connect with.

Connections with loss through the symbolism of mythological and other three-dimensional works of art is not necessarily a process of sexual substitution. As stated in the Introduction to this book, I do not pursue the sexual connotations of lost and found objects in line with Freud's theory of castration and the Oedipus complex (Freud 2010, pp. 280, 376, 379). I leave the deeply personal significance of loss and absence to the individual reader and focus instead on the healing properties of the actual search. I do, however, contend that Freud's work on loss has far more to do with death than with sex; he regarded mourning as the constant work of psy-chotherapy (Burke 2006, p. 143). At times mourning becomes pathologically self-destructive where a type of murder is enacted upon the self or other (Black 2011). The compulsion of Thanatos in the death drive can be counterbalanced through a powerful resurrection of Eros as life-giving. In this way the fetish can also be a wonderful symbol for rising above and sublimating the dying self back into life.

Paranoiac critical method of transference

Before proceeding to the practical part of this chapter, I'd like to bring the process of sublimation and fetishism together with a discussion of the work of twentieth-century Surrealist artist Salvador Dali. Dali's paranoiac critical method is illus-trated here to exemplify approaches that can be used in Section B. There is the dream object, and there is the object in the real world that holds dream qualities.

Both can be used to substitute loss and often the process is one of extended sub-limation where one transcends present reality because it is too painful. Although sceptical of the long-term results of substituting art for loss, Freud (1963, p. 17) wrote that he underwent sublimation with his own art objects but also in the presence of powerful art in the museums of Vienna and Rome (Freud 1963, p. 16; Burke 2006). Therefore paranoia (madness) and critique (rationality) combine when one can concretise profound loss into an object and thereby continue to function in the world. The loss is transferred but also contained and engaged with in the form of artworks, art making, art appreciation and art criticism.

Dali's dream-like landscapes have pieces of mechanical materialism (such as clocks) which are rendered organic and subject to decay to the extent that ants can devour these timepieces. These double realities are represented In Dali's *The Persistence of Memory* (1931). In this painting the strange form in the central brown space that seems to be without gravity is a Daliesque face; when you look at its profile it becomes recognisable. The theme of time as a human construct and object of reality are mocked. Dali indulged in the unreal and was able to bring on voluntary hallucinations, after which he painted in a manic way aided by his remarkable *trompe l'oeil* (photo real) method (Finkelstein 1979, p. 30). The convincing effect of the *trompe l'oeil* is perhaps the most disconcerting aspect of Dali's work; the objects lost, found, altered and also out of place, are rendered hyper-real in technicolour. And when coupled with his paranoiac critical method the image and its objects are given a kind of 'logic' (Finkelstein 1979, p. 30).

The paranoiac critical method can be described as painting something that resembles (usually) two different things, the forms are pictorially manipulated to be reversible. Dali's method of paranoiac criticism is a central method of unlocking the unconscious both in interpreting a work of art and in making one. Despite Dali's admiration for Freud, his use of the term 'paranoia' in this method is not scientific. As mentioned above, Dali was able to simulate a state of paranoia (without drugs) in order to access hallucinatory imagery; he then painted the images which he referred to as hand-painted dream photographs.

Finkelstein (1979) says that paranoiac criticism is 'not merely a technique', adding that it is a manner of 'accommodating reality and its objects to one's own desires and obsessions' (Finkelstein 1979, p. 30). Dali also used Lacan's work on 'paranoid psychosis' but instead of insisting on Lacan's 'meaningfulness of the delusions', Dali promoted the enjoyment of nonsense (Levine 2008, p. 76). Both Dali and André Breton developed their own versions of the paranoiac critical in art. In this context Surrealism and its art take what they need from the layers of the unconscious and deliberately mix them up in the conscious. For example, what might look distinctly like a face to one person is something entirely different to another depending on her/his state of consciousness at the time, or, to be more specific, depending on what their current fetish might be. In the paranoiac critical method of painting there is a conscious manipulation on the part of the artist but it also opens doors to the unconscious for the viewer. Therefore the 'paranoid' part is the muddling of realities and the 'critical' part is the interpretation of those realities. The object asserts itself via the paranoiac critical method's activity. The Surrealists admired the dream world but 'did not wish to remain asleep in it' (Foster 1995, p. 163).

Section B: Practical: the unconscious and healing practices

Once again, as you approach the exercises, take time to check in with yourself before you embark on the searching that is integral to all the processes that follow. Return to some of the mindfulness techniques in Chapters 1 and 3 of this book to settle yourself if necessary.

Locating pain: Monica's lost and found objects

Pain in this context is emotional pain; however, it's important to remember that physical symptoms are often related to extreme emotional stress. The dream material presented here is a result of several connected dreams that initially are a strong play of opposites. Monica was aware of the difference between latent and manifest dream content and when processing her dreams she put her efforts into bringing the absent into the present. In the first dream of the sequence, the manifest content is the sleeping wolf-dog; however, Monica knew there was something else in that darkness which had not yet taken on a precise form or texture. She felt the space 'it' used up and the shape of that space began to become apparent. Because of the initial lack of detailed information from the unconscious, but intent on not losing that which was available, Monica chose to cut the shape out of a different piece of paper and superimpose it beside the dog. The shape at this stage of retrieval does not have substance (form, texture, identity) but it extends beyond the boundaries of the represented dream space (Figure 5.1). Monica is

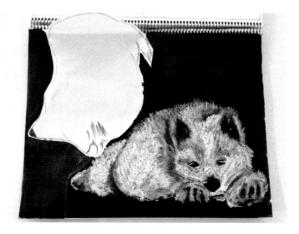

FIGURE 5.1   *Monica's Sleeping Dog and Shape* (2014), collage, charcoal, pencil and acrylic in an art journal.

Reproduced in accordance with ethics protocols.

well on the way to locating and acknowledging her pain. Before this it was kept in the darkness of her unconscious; now she courageously opens the door.

The dream text for this sequence of Monica's dreams is restricted to single words or short phrases and is not a running narrative. The words float in the space of her journal beside repeated line drawings of a flower design. Repetition is used to reinforce what is now evident as a recurring dream, but at this stage the relationship between the dog, the 'shape' and the flower designs are not clear. The floating dream words include: 'scars', 'brain surgery', 'let the monsters see you smile', 'security blanket' and family names in the petals of one flower design. Monica also pastes sections from Freud's *Interpretation of Dreams* into her journal. One selected quote is:

> Dreams feel themselves at liberty, moreover, to represent any element by its wishful contrary; so there is no way of deciding at a first glance whether any element that admits of a contrary is present in the dream-thoughts as a positive or as a negative.
>
> *(Freud 2010, p. 334)*

Another quote Monica included after finally representing her dream object (Figure 5.2) is:

> Touch brings solidity to the dream. Touch honors another energy in a very intimate way. Wild dreams tell us that everything in creation has been touched in a special way and that through touch in our dreams, we will remember ourselves as women of power.
>
> *(Kaplan 2000, p. 154)*

Monica diligently worked through all related dreams to locate her pain and find an object that could both represent the pain but also provide healing. She

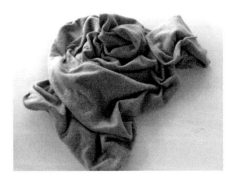

FIGURE 5.2 *Monica's Dream Object: Blanket with Stitching* (2014), fleece and cotton stitching.

Reproduced in accordance with ethics protocols.

arrived at the soft-textured blanket (Figure 5.2) by linking the fur on the dog with the flat shape in that dream. This link provided the missing texture and form which is protective and comforting. Making such connections is only possible in dreamwork analysis (Freud 2010). The flower design representing her family is subtly stitched into the blanket with barely visible white running stitches. The blanket itself reminds her of being close to death, confronting what might be on the other side of this life, and being fearful of recurring symptoms. The 'monster' is the anxiety associated with this fear and the 'scars' are shared by her family who also provide Monica with 'security'.

This brings us to the end of Monica's dreamwork and provides preparatory information for the healing practices that follow.

Exercises

Your own lost objects: a dream journal exercise

Materials: dream journal; collage materials, objects in your home/studio/office.

- Ensure that you are psychologically prepared to locate your pain. You might not know it's there or precisely where it is, when it will return, or what form it will take.
- As with previous chapters, now is the time to consult your own dream journal as a resource. Using Monica's dream as an example might help you link apparently unconnected dreams and dream images.
- Search into the dream representations for what is not there and identify what is there as a possible representation of its opposite. This inversion can assist in locating points of pain to slowly arrive at what could be an object that contains the pain.
- Make a collage of connected dreams and dream images as a creative way of dealing with the messages that your unconscious provides.
- Pay careful attention to the amount of space objects take up and notice the 'negative space' between representations carefully. Additional work on negative space is covered in the next exercise.
- When you have completed your collage, spend time with it and honour it as a map of your pain with clues on managing it. At this stage it may be that you are inspired to make another artwork, perhaps something in three dimensions like a clay pot, an embroidered cushion or a painted stone. These objects will be more than ornaments for you; they will be memorials to your suffering and a testimony to your strength, so choose the form and materials that give you comfort.

Or (existing objects in your home/studio/office):

- Alternatively there may already be a tangible object or objects in your personal spaces that you acquired and which have a certain presence.

- These could be art objects that you look at and they might be objects that seem to look at you; either way they will be objects that draw you to them.
- Choose one object at a time.
- Consider what its essence might be.
- What is it saying to you? Jean Martin Charcot, the neurologist that Freud studied under at Salpétrière in Paris, gave the following advice to Freud: 'look at the same things again and again until they themselves begin to speak' (Burke 2006, p. 155).
- Does the object and its message or implied meaning have any connection to any of the images in your dream journal?
- Reflect on what is communicated across your conscious (your room and your chosen object) and unconscious spaces (your dream journal).
- Sit with that communication and, if you feel the need, develop one of your dream journal images incorporating your found object even further. This could be a painting or another medium of your choice.

In the collage, painting or other art form, a degree of sublimation should take place if you allow yourself the space, and if you work in a good temenos (see Chapter 3 for setting up a temenos).

Paranoiac critical method

Explanation

This is a method that Salvador Dali developed but the concept of seeing at least two distinct forms in one image is ancient. Monks illustrating medieval biblical manuscripts hid all sorts of creatures in their illustrations of religious stories; sometimes these came from pagan themes which is why they were disguised in the Catholic monasteries. More recently (1899) but still earlier than Dali, the Polish-born American psychologist Joseph Jastrow used the cartoon of a 'duck – rabbit' (Figure 5.3) to point out that perception is both visual and mental. Another example, *The Rubin Vase* devised by Danish psychologist Edgar John Rubin in 1915 (Figure 5.4), uses a simple silhouette technique. An important part of the paranoiac critical method is the use of so-called negative space; this is the space between objects but for our purposes it is anything by negative – it has its own form and is therefore charged with positivity.

When looking sideways at the *African Village Postcard* (Figure 5.6), which inspired Salvador Dali's oil painting, *Paranoiac Village* (1931), a three-quarter profile becomes apparent. For example, the dark forms of the three centrally seated figures become the space beneath the nose, and the definition of the mouth and chin. The left eye and cheek are formed by the recumbent figure and the right eye is formed by the merged dark group of seated figures. See Figures 5.5 and 5.6. The result of this sideways view takes on the style of the early phase of Analytical Cubist painting when objects were still recognisable and not entirely

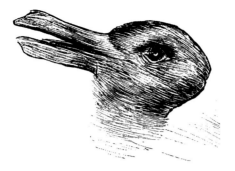

FIGURE 5.3 Joseph Jastrow (1899), *Duck–Rabbit*, pencil drawing based on the original unattributed cartoon from 23 October 1892 issue of *Fliegende Blätter* (Fugitive Sheets), a German satirical weekly.

In the public domain, copyright expired.

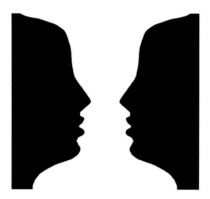

FIGURE 5.4 Edgar Rubin (1915), *The Rubin Vase*, ink on paper. Creative Commons CC–by-sa 3.0 License (CC-by-sa).

In the public domain.

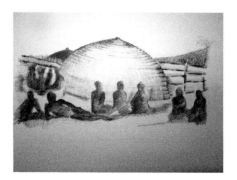

FIGURE 5.5 Kathleen Connellan (2018), coloured pencil drawing copy of *African Village postcard*.

In the public domain.

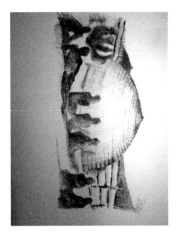

FIGURE 5.6 Kathleen Connellan (2018), coloured pencil drawing copy of *African Village postcard* side view.

In the public domain.

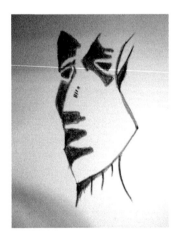

FIGURE 5.7 Kathleen Connellan (2018), coloured pencil drawing of *African Village postcard* with a Dali face.

Author's own artwork.

abstracted (Figure 5.7). However Dali adapted the scene using his own more realistic surreal style of painting, making the profile look like his wife Gala's face in a typically Daliesque manner. This was the beginning of the Surrealists' paranoiac critical method.

Materials: pencils, pens and inks. Acrylic paint, stretched canvas or thick card for developed works.

Process:

- Observe something in nature that has interesting spaces between its forms; for example, cloud formations, vine leaves, patterns in sand.
- Photograph those that appear to have forms within forms, where you might see faces, figures or objects. Print the photographs.
- On a piece of paper transfer (draw or trace) the visual perception of the photographed images so that the double identity is clear to you but might not be immediately clear to others.
- Another method of transferring the photographed forms is to cut the dominant forms out in black paper paying careful attention to edge detail (use small sharp scissors), then place the black shapes onto white paper. This will create silhouettes and allow the white spaces between to come forward and assume their own recognisable shapes.

Or:

- Consult you dream journal and look for dreams that have 'negative' space that could be something else that you had not previously observed. This is a way of looking into the void and finding that it is anything but empty.
- Another way of finding presence in absence is to turn the dream images in your dream journal around slowly looking at them sideways and upside down. What do you see?
- Prepare a canvas or piece of card of a size that suits you and pencil in the drawing from your dream journal.
- Choose appropriate colours carefully and in tune with your emotions so that you are able to paint a scene that has hidden figures and objects in one view or becomes a completely different scene when viewed upside down or sideways.
- While you are in the process, try not to force one thing to be another; let the forms naturally evolve from what you saw and sensed in the space and which has specific meaning for you. What you're doing is developing the objet-imago as a conduit from the preconscious to the conscious from your dream.
- Consider what symbolic content the objet-imago has for you. What emotions does it hold? Does it help locate grief, pain, ecstasy, anger, fear, doubt or other emotions?
- Sit with your emotions, notice where they might resonate in your body as you engage with your artwork.
- In your own time make a promise to yourself that will help care for that pain or other significant emotions.

Exquisite corpse (group work)

This is a collaborative and intuitive technique used by the Surrealists.

Hints for group work: Irvin Yalom (1975) provides some excellent benefits for the therapeutic benefits of group work. These include: the curative effects of trust; instillation of hope; universality (one is not alone); relationship skills; unconditional positive regard; altruism; information giving; corrective recapitulation of primary family (role strengthening that mirror healthy family units); improved social skills; imitative positive behaviour; interpersonal learning; group cohesiveness; catharsis; existential openness to discuss fears and challenges such as death (Yalom 1975, pp. 2, 3). Bear in mind that conflict is a natural element in group work with humans. Yalom writes that 'conflict can be harnessed to service the group' (1975, p. 352). For example, the composite group image might end up being a strange conglomeration of creatures, humans, objects, natural forms and imaginary forms. The contradictions and conflicts will be always already there and this is what makes for richness in imaginative arts practice. Accepting difference amongst each other in the group is therefore an important aspect whilst acknowledging that conflict is an indication of something unresolved within ourselves that can be worked upon.

A popular way to sum up the benefits of group work is 'forming, norming, storming, performing and mourning' (Tuckman 1965). These all allow for hidden objects to form and to render them normal by realising that others have the same or similar issues; also to face them head on together, take time to reflect, adjourn and if necessary grieve together. It's good to have a group leader but this role should be gentle so that group norms can be established and not viewed as 'rules' but rather as a consensus for the activity. One important norm should be confidentiality; therefore the result of the final image and how it is shared is important to establish at the start.

Materials: one long piece of paper that is folded like a concertina and which can open out at the end to show all contributions in one. Graphite pencil or black pen. White chalk pastel on black paper is also effective and was used by the Surrealists, Valentino Hugo, André Breton and Tristan Tzara in *Landscape: The Exquisite Corpse*, 1933, chalk on paper (Chipp 1968, p. 419).

Process:

- Fold the paper into sufficient sections for everyone and ensure all present understand the following process.
- Everyone should have some idea of what their objet–imago looks like in their mind.
- When one person is drawing, others should not watch.
- One person starts with a drawing of their objet-imago allowing just the lines on the bottom edge of the drawing to overlap into the very top of the next section, fold the drawing back and pass the paper to the next person.
- The next person draws their object-imago joining onto the lines at the top of their section, also letting the lines at the bottom of their drawing overlap into the next section of folded paper.
- Fold the drawing back and pass the paper to the next person.

- Continue until everyone has had a turn.
- Return the folded paper to the group leader who opens it out and spreads the extended drawing on the table for everyone to reflect upon.

Reflection

Share what has emerged and discuss this in turn and as a group:

(a) Brainstorm the composite image; note commonalities and differences in your discussion. Address seemingly shocking aspects by being completely un-judgemental and allowing everyone unconditional positive regard to share their reflections.
(b) Photograph/record the composite image for future use and further reflection and/or artistic developed work.
(c) Allow ample time to acknowledge sorrow and to plan for joy that will come from additional self-knowledge and care.

Conclusion

This chapter has tried to settle upon the object and hear what it has to say. However, as the discussion on sublimation and substitution has shown, the object is often not recognised for what it symbolises; additionally an object can be fetishised to cope with loss. Sections of the chapter demonstrate that the object can enter our consciousness uninvited but its absence can also create a void. Therefore there can be a crisis of longing if the object is not where it is needed.

The chapter shows that in Freudian and Lacanian terms, absence represents a lack and for our purposes dream analysis becomes a place for discovering what lies at the root of loss. One might not even know what is lost, but in dreams lack is often central; it might be the lack of an ending, destination or resolution because dreams are almost always incomplete. Therefore by using dream theory, the lost object can be found through representations of dreams which are processed appropriately by the viewer or artist or both. Loss can be the loss of something/someone but also, and significantly, it can be the loss of something more abstract, like hope, security or love. For example, Lacan posited that the smile of Leonardo da Vinci's *Mona Lisa*, 1517, oil on wood panel, represented the artist's lost maternal love (Levine 2008). Monica's sleeping dog in this chapter represents the comfort and strength that she had in her childhood but needed to reclaim.

However, there is enormous therapeutic benefit in having fun and not taking all objects in the unconscious too seriously. Much can be discovered through relaxing and playing with images as Dali has shown. Dali (1935) believed in representing paranoia for itself. Therefore we have the object as a point of analysis but the entire painting's uncanny mixture can be a necessary non-sense. The non-sense is a commentary on many personal dilemmas but can also be a profound method for parody. For example, Dali's paintings frequently parodied the pointlessness of war and the madness of power during the 1930s in Europe. Dali's Surrealistic *trompe l'oeil* method seemed to give the dream object a concreteness therefore providing a more defined point of departure in the analysis.

The exercises in Section B such as the dream journal work, using the paranoiac-critical and exquisite corpse methods, all help to find the lost object and recognise it for our process of healing. In conducting these exercises as a therapeutic process, it's possible to translate the abstract object into one with more clarity. In the words of Yalom (1975, p. 134), 'The therapist moves the focus from outside to inside, from abstract to the specific, from the generic to the personal'.

Notes

1 This chapter owes its title to the published PhD thesis of H.N. Finkelstein (1979), *Surrealism and the Crisis of the Object*, University of Michigan Press, Ann Arbor, MI.
2 Hal Foster (1992) provides clarity on the three main understandings of fetish: the anthropological, the Marxian and the Freudian.

References

Black, D.M. (2011), *Why Things Matter: The place of values in science, psychoanalysis and religion*, Routledge, London.

Burke, J. (2006), *The Gods of Freud: Sigmund Freud's art collection*, Knopf, Sydney.

Caws, M.A. (2011), 'Meret Oppenheim's Fur Teacup', *Gastronomica*, vol. 11, no. 3, pp. 25–28.

Chipp, H.B. (1968), *Theories of Modern Art: A source book artists and critics*, University of California Press, Los Angeles.

Dali, S. (1935), *Conquest of the Irrational*, trans. D. Gascoyne, Julien Levy, New York.

de Botton, A. and Armstrong, J. (2013), *Art as Therapy*, Phaidon, London.

Finkelstein, H.N. (1979), *Surrealism and the Crisis of the Object*, University of Michigan Press, Ann Arbor, MI.

Finkelstein, J. (2010), 'Fashioned Identity and the Unreliable Image', *Critical Studies in Fashion and Beauty*, vol. 1, no. 2, pp. 161–171.

Foster, H. (1992), 'The Art of Fetishism', in *Fetish: The Princeton Architectural Journal*, vol. 4, pp. 6–19.

Foster, H. (1995), *Compulsive Beauty*, MIT Press, Cambridge, MA.

Freud, S. (1927), *The Complete Psychological Works of Sigmund Freud: Vol. XXI*, trans. J Strachey, Hogarth Press and Institute of Psychoanalysis, London.

Freud, S. (1963), *Civilization and its Discontents*, trans. J. Riviere, rev. edn, Hogarth Press and Institute of Psychoanalysis, London.

Freud, S. (2010), *The Interpretation of Dreams*, trans. J. Strachey, Basic Books, New York.

Jung, C.G. (2002), *Dreams*, trans. R.F.C. Hull, Routledge, London.

Kaplan, C.C. (2000), *The Woman's Book of Dreams: Dreaming as a spiritual practice*, Beyond Words Publishing, Hillsboro, OR.

Lacan, J. (2006), *Écrits*, trans. B. Fink, Norton, London.

Levine, S.Z. (2008), *Lacan Reframed*, Tauris, London.

Lippard, L.R. (1970), *Surrealists on Art*, Allen & Unwin, Englewood Cliffs, NJ.

Lippard, L.R. (1997), *Six Years: The dematerialisation of the art object*, University of California Press, Los Angeles.

Symons, J.M. (2016), 'Ambiguity Makes Sense: An Exploration of the Creative Relationship between Mothering and Painting; Featuring Contemporary Oil Painting Practice as an Auto-Ethnographic Research Methodology', PhD thesis, University of South Australia, Adelaide.

Tuckman, B.W. (1965), 'Developmental Sequence in Small Groups', *Psychological Bulletin*, vol. 63, no. 6, pp. 334–399.

Yalom, I.D. (1975), *The Theory and Practice of Group Psychotherapy*, 2nd edn, Basic Books, New York.

6

SENSORY TRIGGERS[1]

Beyond sight

Introduction

The visual sense has assumed a privileged status in the Western imaginary particularly since the seventeenth-century French philosopher René Descartes influenced the mind/body split. Under this Cartesian philosophy the eye became the eye of the mind, and the body was relegated to the lower messy region of the sinful senses. Cartesian separation is still employed by some but it is widely accepted that consistent division of the mind and body is unhealthy. In dreaming, healing and imaginative arts practice, bodily senses such as sound, scent, texture and taste add substantially to recollection, which in turn compensates for loss. As such this chapter builds on Chapter 5 by showing that the imagined or real object is only partially understood by the sense of sight. The aim of this chapter is to move beyond sight into the physical body as a primary site of perception. A secondary aim is to show that the senses of the body are not only connected to each other but also to what is outside the body in the material world. Therefore a phenomenological approach is taken to situate the body (our body) amongst other bodies (including substances and matter), and to gain more insight from their relationships and shared perceptions.

Once again the chapter is divided into theory and practice. Section A, the theoretical section that is located in our conscious state, reviews writings on all the senses sequentially even though they are connected. I begin with the olfactory senses of taste and smell, moving on to the sense of touch, followed by sound and ending with sight. The writers I draw from include key figures such as Marcel Proust (2006), Maurice Merleau-Ponty (2002) and Hal Foster (1988). Section B, the practical section, recounts an art therapy project I conducted in an aged care facility where three men and three women, all in various stages of dementia, made a collage of their memories based predominantly on touch, taste and sound. This is provided as a case study and an example for retrieving old memories with the body, not the mind. The exercises that follow the case study use collaged art forms of mixed media, sound and movement. Materials privilege tactile sensory qualities. Images are included to inspire and show that collage need not only be in relief but can also be three dimensional and susceptible to air moving through it to capture dreams.

Section A: Theory: conscious reflections on the senses

The olfactory senses: taste and smell

Simon Schama (1995) begins *Landscape and Memory* with this epigrammatic quote from Henry David Thoreau (1856): 'It is in vain to dream of a wildness distant from ourselves. There is none such. It is the bog in our brains and bowels, the primitive vigor of Nature in us, that inspires that dream' (Schama 1995, p. 7). With this in mind, let us move straight to the stomach, the engine room of our bodies. There are several sayings currently used to connect the stomach to one's emotions, thoughts and actions. Some include: 'I feel it in my pit/gut/insides' or 'I have butterflies in my stomach' or 'my stomach churns at the thought' or 'it was a gut response' or 'she's got guts (intestinal fortitude)'or 'it leaves a bad taste' and others besides. The stomach is a site for processing but the material processed is quite easily visualised as messy matter; therefore to align it with thinking is to taint the purity of thought *if* one believes the Cartesian trope. In the medieval monastic culture, long before Descartes, the Latin term '*ruminatio*' was used for prayers because this soul thinking was regarded as the ruminating of images (Carruthers 2007, p. 51). To ruminate is a wonderful term that has more embodiment than its counterpart verb, 'to reflect'. Mary Carruthers writes, 'Reading is to be digested, to be ruminated, like a cow chewing her cud, or like a bee making honey from the nectar of flowers' (2007, p. 51). In dreaming, healing and imaginative arts practice, we are not necessarily talking about reading; the process for us is closer to the medieval monastic process of ruminating dream imagery. The stomach is also a site of memory because in the process of 'regurgitation', 'the stored texts [images] are the sweet-smelling cud originally drawn from the meadows of books [dreams], they are chewed in the palate' (Carruthers 2007, p. 51). Carruthers refers to these and other digestive metaphors as a way of 'domesticating' something and making it our own (2007, p. 55).

Taking something into one's body is often as a result of an arousal from its aroma, followed shortly by its taste. Ede (2013, p. xiv) notes that the olfactory system is our most primitive sense (Ede 2013, p. xiv), and Hillman calls smell the 'undersense' (1979, p. 187); it is what alerts the animal in us to both danger and pleasure. Additionally Ede points out that the olfactory system has no links to those parts of the brain responsible for language or speech which she says might explain why it is so difficult to find words to describe smell directly and without analogy. Smell in dreams is rare but Hillman says that when they do occur they signify an 'intense psychic acuity to discern' the 'nature' of the dream object, adding that 'when we smell something, we are taking in its spirit (Hillman 1979, p. 187). Section B will explore sensory associations and analogies as a means of capturing essence.

It is impossible to talk about the sensory delights of scent and taste without referring to the legendary text by Proust in his *À la recherche du temps perdu* (2006). Proust had returned home from a dull day at work; it was a cold evening so his mother offered him a cup of tea and a madeleine. At first sip his mind and body flooded with a sublime but anguished sensation for a lost childhood memory, which, after searching for it by 'clearing a space in front' of his mind (2006, p. 62), he recounted with extraordinary precision:

> And once I had recognized the taste of the crumb of madeleine soaked in her decoction of lime-flowers which my aunt used to give me . . . immediately the old grey house upon the street, where her room was, rose up like the scenery of a theatre to attach itself to the little pavilion, opening on to the garden . . . so in that moment all the flowers in our garden and in [the] park, and the water-lilies on the Vivonne and the good folk of the village and their little dwellings and the parish church and the whole of Combray and its surroundings, taking their proper shapes and growing solid, sprang into being, town and gardens alike, from my cup of tea.
>
> *(2006, p. 63)*

This taste memory brought joy to Proust but scents and associated tastes can also recall sadness, unpleasant and even dangerous experiences. Remaining with poetic prose for the moment, it is possible that the pungent smell of ripe fruit would remind the poet Christina Rossetti (if she was writing about herself) of the fruit she ate from the fabled goblin's market. She traded a golden lock of her hair to taste their enticing fruit:

> Sweeter than honey from the rock, Stronger than man-rejoicing wine, Clearer than water flowed that juice; She never tasted such before, . . . She sucked and sucked the more, Fruits which that unknown orchard bore; She sucked until her lips were sore.
>
> *(Rossetti 1996, p. 27, 28)*

Drinking the 'sugar-sweet . . . sap' and biting into 'peaches with a velvet nap' amongst other fruits resulted in constant unrequited longing that brought decline and gradual death to the girl in Rossetti's poem (Rossetti 1996, p. 29). These delicious and forbidden fruits have both flavour and texture; therefore with the surfaces of desire and longing in mind let us move to the sense of touch.

Touch

Touch is the sense that calls us to reach out from our bodies to touch another, signalling a need and commitment to engage. Merleau-Ponty (2002) writes about the exploratory engagement of touch that extends passive sight into action, 'like the exploratory gaze of true vision, the knowing touch projects us outside our body through movement' (Merleau-Ponty 2002, p. 367). Touch's seeking can be tentative: 'my hand moves around the object it touches, anticipating the stimuli and itself tracing out the form I am about to perceive' (Merleau-Ponty 2002, p. 87). There is also daring in touch; it is the ultimate connection with another, crossing the divide and creating a union. Throughout history touch has been held as the 'fundamental source of information to integrate the senses' (Wade 2013, p. 25). Touch breaks down the Cartesian division of the senses and forces us to form organic thoughts where the psychic and the physiological are one (Merleau-Ponty 2002, p. 89).

However touch can also be unsettling, and has 'the potential to subvert the hierarchical relationship between object and beholder' (Johnson 2013, p. 77). Touch does not work one way, it is reciprocal, and as such it can disturb power relations which is why touch should also be used with caution and respect. Touch can be destructive and violate respected distance; therefore whilst it is sensual it also holds the horror of violence in this disturbing ambiguity at its disposal.

Touch is also often referred to as a means of verifying information; the famous biblical example is the Risen Christ inviting the doubting disciple Thomas to put his fingers into the crucifixion wounds in his side and hands (John 20:24–29). Seeing is not necessarily believing, and now in our increasingly technologised world touch is neutralised on a flat touch screen and becomes mechanical. For touch to 'work' in an integrative way with all the senses, texture, sound, smell and the visual are all important components.

Sound

Sound and scent are closely related and often precede touch. Sounds, like scents, alerts us to both peril and pleasure. Both are primeval, even animal; the physicist Brian Cox (2015) informs us that the evolution of sound is so old that it developed below water before reaching the air above when the earth's masses were formed. Cox (2015) refers to sound in the dark depths of underwater caves as the setting for the fine tuning of this primordial sense. Those depth sounds existed and exist in their own time, not the time of rushed human life. When tuning into sound memories and listening to melodic or other inspirational sounds, one can borrow a kind of deep listening from the ocean depths. Susan Tomes (2014) tells that it is important to listen slowly; to be in a time-space that is not a short sequence but something enduring that one can rest into and regain oneself. For example Tuan (1977) writes that 'sounds greatly enrich the human feeling of space' (1977, p. 14). Tuan cites musicologist Roberto Gerhard as saying 'form in music means knowing at every moment exactly where one is. Consciousness of form is really a sense of orientation' (Tuan 1977, p. 15).

This powerful sense of sound and particularly musical sound, is said to be the most enduring cognitive enhancer in dementia patients (Baird and Samson 2015; Stevens 2015). Music is sound organised in a certain way (Sadie 1986). For dreaming, healing and imaginative arts practice, music is a beautifully symbolic way of inscribing memories. Merleau-Ponty writes, 'sound leads to content' (2002, p. 31) – it can return knowledges and narratives back into an expression of self.

> sounds once perceived can be followed only by other sounds, or by silence, which is not an auditory nothingness, but the absence of sounds, and which, therefore, keeps us in contact with the being of sound. If, during the process of reflections, I cease to hear sounds, and then suddenly become receptive to them again, they appear to me to be already there, and I pick up a thread which I had dropped but which is unbroken.
>
> *(Merleau-Ponty 2002, pp. 382, 383)*

Merleau-Ponty emphasises silence as an important component of sound. Living in an urban area, there is no real silence and even then the sounds may be rendered as noise. If a quiet space can be found and especially if one is out in the desert or in a remote piece of nature, then the true harmonies of silence can be heard. Section B will develop practices of silence by bringing sounds of silence and of music inside the body, uniting them with the spirit in a state of being. This is what Merleau-Ponty calls the ontology of sound; it is where the body and sound allow transcendence of space to occur.

Sight

I have left sight to last because, as I said in the introduction, it is given too much emphasis to the detriment of the other senses. However, I'd like to take vision and turn it inside out, so that inverted vision becomes a 'visuality' that 'involves the body and the psyche' (Foster 1988, p. ix). Foster (1995) draws on Walter Benjamin (1968) to develop his ideas on visuality. For Benjamin, the dream world and inner vision is 'auratic'. In this way the aura of the artist's body and spirit link the inner and outer eye (Benjamin 1968). As such visuality is deeper and clearer than vision, the mind's eye 'dilates with surprise and joy' in the dark of the psyche (Hillman 1979, p. 191). Vision is too crowded: 'Sight says too many things at one time (Bachelard 1994, p. 215). Vision is also socially and historically situated and is too often divorced from other senses. Visuality, on the other hand, is truer to the body and less of a slave to the opinions of others. John Berger's famous text on *Ways of Seeing* (1972) is testimony to the influence of social hierarchies and representations in visual culture that affect the way we see ourselves. Berger (1972), followed by Bryson (1988), developed the notion of the gaze and the returning gaze in art and visual culture. Additionally, generations of feminists critique the male gaze for constructing the woman as an object and subjecting her to male dominance. Furthermore post-colonial studies adopt a similar critique to feminism where racial dominance is interrogated through a revision of racial supremacy. All these scholars build on Foucault's work on the medical gaze first published in France in 1963 where the body is the subject of medical scrutiny and is at risk of losing independence from the 'penetrating gaze' of the physician (Foucault 1994, p. 15). Lacan took Foucault's work in a different direction and applied the gaze (*le regard*) in his theory of the mirrored self. So it was not just how others (like those in authority) see us but how we see ourselves in them. This is known as the Lacanian 'mirror stage' when the ego of the child first enters the language of society, recognises itself in others and may begin to emulate them (Levine 2008).

With the above theories in mind, it is easy to understand how the dominance of sight can distort our inner balance and even rob us of a sense of bodily self. The social world and technological worlds can be machines of surveillance with eyes everywhere so that we lose our inner visuality and risk being split in many ways. Section B sets exercises, first, to strengthen the inner eye as a means of re-knowing and caring for ourselves; and, second, to develop a reciprocal gaze so that we as subjects of others' gazes can withstand scrutiny or return love as appropriate.

Section B: Practical: the unconscious and healing practices

Case study: senses of memory

The setting is a residential aged care facility with a closed dementia unit. It is a beautifully designed home with leafy gardens, water features, 'almost' real animals in the shrubs and dedicated staff. I was fortunate to be able to work with three gentlemen and three ladies, all with varying stages of dementia. Each of them made a piece of collage like a slice of pizza which then fitted together into a large circle. However, for the purposes of brevity, I'll concentrate on the input of one gentleman who I'll call Eric and one lady who I'll call Daisy. The university I worked for and the facility concerned granted ethics approval for publication of material from this sensory arts therapy project called 'Senses of Memory'.

Eric

The first time I met Eric he was in his 'shed'. The door of his bedroom in the closed unit has a bright handmade sign proclaiming 'Eric's Shed' with an image of a shed on it. In Australia, a shed in the backyard is a (usually male) domain linked to hobbies and outdoor jobs. Eric appeared physically quite strong and certainly not elderly. He was dead keen to get involved in making a collage of his memories and we started with a lively conversation about his favourite foods, music and experiences. From this first meeting I gathered that he loved oats porridge because it gave him the energy he needed for the long bush walks he went on with his mates, and he also loved to sing whilst he walked. The second time I arrived with a bag of Australian lemon-gum (*eucoeucalyptus citriodora*) leaves and pods, bright parrot feathers, music recordings, life-like images of Australian birds and bush animals, mouth-watering images of steaming oats porridge (I couldn't take food in) and a few other articles so we could begin his collage. Eric wasn't in his 'shed' and after searching around I discovered him in a jaunty cap, pushing his walker equipped with binoculars, camera, a water bottle and some other odds and ends as if he was really on one of his long walks. He was humming and smiling and quite a favourite with the ladies. We went to his shed where he joyfully engaged in selecting, cutting and gluing his collage together (Figure 6.1). Recollecting further he remembered the magpies and was positively gleeful when I played a recording of the Australian magpie's warbling song. After a moment he also broke into song with his whole body moving in rhythm to 'Alexander's Rag Time Band'. Significantly, on my next visit when I produced the sheet music for that song including the typed lyrics and a recording, the usually jovial Eric became angry. I quickly put the words out of sight and, regaining his cheer, Eric listened to recordings and sang along. By offering him the visual coded language of writing, I was robbing him of what he had preciously retained. He could still remember the words and desperately needed to keep them in his body and mind.

Daisy

Entering Daisy's room was like going into a magical cave. Daisy sat in a chair in a far corner with the dappled light of a large garden window shining on her pearly white hair. Her voice rang out to me like a lute in the wind; she seemed quite ethereal. Daisy had filled her room with glittering objects. When I approached she was making jewellery with sparkling beads, to add to her adornment (Figure 6.2).

She invited me to sit on the lace cover of the bed beside her chair and we began our explorative conversations to identify and match art materials that resonated with Daisy's sensory capacities: What were her favourite foods as a child and younger woman? What were some of the textures she could remember

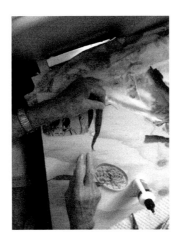

FIGURE 6.1 Kathleen Connellan (2014), *Eric Preparing His Collage.*

Author's own photograph.

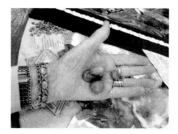

FIGURE 6.2 Kathleen Connellan (2014), *Daisy's Rings, Bracelets and Pebbles.*
Author's own photograph.

touching and feeling? Did she have any songs or tunes she loved to recall? Asking such questions of Daisy was like opening up a sensory opera. She grew up in London in the war and post-war years and remembered eating jellied eels from Smithfield Market, and having mushy peas with faggots.

> Nice mash potatoes with eels, I had them all my life in England, ooh yummy . . .
> and the pease pudding and faggots we used to have that on a Sunday, you
> see . . . Oh and I remember the velvet dress I used to wear to church on
> Sundays too . . . red velvet with a white lace collar with little pink roses . . .
> I had another one the same . . . blue . . . my favourite colour is red . . . . and
> yes, I remember walking barefoot on the pebbled beach.
>
> *(interview data, 2014)*

I had no shortage of information and came laden with velvet, lace, sea sand, shells, pebbles, song recordings, nutmeg and other herbs and spices from the recipes, including realistic images of favourite foods. Daisy attacked the task of collaging with zest. The urgency to put the collage together became palpable, Daisy's states of consciousness fluctuated as if the preconscious was speaking to her and activating her body, and at times she sang her special songs whilst in the art process. It was with intensity that Daisy cut fabric and paper, pasted, coloured with thick oily pastel creating a beach scene, stroked the velvet, embroidered pink flowers onto lace, wrote out the recipe for jellied eels, and attached nutmegs and dried herbs whilst absorbing their fragrance. All of this she collated, curated and collaged into a composite life story. At times, during the process, Daisy was totally immersed in the materials. When I cautiously checked in with her (not wanting to interrupt her state of consciousness) and asked where or how she was, looking up to my face with her fingers in the sand, shells and thick pastel, she replied, 'I'm here on the beach but I can't tell you how I feel, there are no words' (interview data). See Plates 19 and 20 in the colour-plate section at the back of the book.

Daisy, Eric and the other four residents involved in the collage held onto themselves and the bits of their life's relationships that were slipping out of reach.

Laying out the objects and materials were like connecting the fragments of past with their present being. When all six came together and witnessed each other's work with amazement whilst joining all pieces together as a whole, it was indeed a sensory performance. Emotions ranged from tears to laughter, with songs and shared stories emanating from the tactile visuality of their collage. Later a 'Lazy Susan' swivel bearing was attached in the centre so that the 1 metre diameter collage could rotate; it was mounted on the wall in one of the lounges (Plate 21 in the colour-plate section).

Exercises

Collaging your dream senses exercise

Materials:

- dream journal with images and notes from nocturnal dreams, daydreams and memories;
- a collection of materials that are manageable to fix onto a surface of your choice – anything from nature or material culture, remnants of your past, symbols of a dreamed future (the choice will be personal so I cannot prescribe);
- good-quality craft glue/a glue gun, and other fixing materials like string, needle and cotton, tacks, stapler, scissors, cutting knife, etc.;
- a durable/tough base substance like wood or thick cardboard, or if you're making a piece of textile art (e.g. Plate 22 in the colour-plate section) your base fabric should be thick cotton drill or denim;
- for a dream catcher: a circular wooden frame or one that you make out of reeds or pliable branches, thick twine, beads, shells (e.g. Plate 23).

Process:

- An alternative term for this exercise is bricolage, which may be even more appropriate as it emphasises the materiality of rediscovered objects and the joys of reshaping and reusing in an existence where sustainability is crucial.
- For the above case study in an aged care home, the sensory materials were collected through careful exploratory conversations, but for you embarking on your own process now, you might only need to *return to your dream journal* which is a treasure trove of sensory reminders.
- Ask yourself these questions when you revisit your dreams: What do/did I smell? What do/did I hear? What does/did it feel like on my skin? What was the temperature in my dream, was I hot or cold, clammy or shivering?

  One of my doctoral students recently shared a dream with me that involved extreme temperature and she generously gave me permission to share it here:

  > I had a dying dream last night. I was in a dark cave partially filled with water, and I was very cold. 'This must be what it's like when you die', I thought (in my dream). Because when you die your body becomes

cold. I became colder and colder until I 'died' but I awoke shivering and relieved to be alive.

Hillman (1979) writes that cave dreams indicate the need for 'loving attention' but that cold in dreams is 'glacial' and cold waters are 'dispassionate' (1979, pp. 151, 152). Admittedly the above dream is chilly in a disturbing way, but very rarely are we able to control nocturnal dreams, whatever their 'temperature'. It's sometimes possible to stay in the dream and pull up another blanket but in my student's case she awoke. If a dream similar to this is in your journal, spend more time in that 'cave', noticing what other sensory responses were present. If one accepts Hillman then the cave of potential warmth and love that is also dripping with glacially cold waters is profoundly and symbolically contradictory.

- Whatever your dream content, gather your materials with 'your eyes wide closed'; imagine you have feelers, heighted hearing, an acute sense of smell and a prickly skin that picks up all around it.
- You may need to go on long walks to practise your sensory responses (see 'Going for a walk and sense harvesting', later in Section B of this chapter).
- Make a list of necessary materials to collect or purchase what your sensory memory and responses have told you.
- You'll know you have sufficient materials to begin your art when you see them altogether in a pile and notice their textural relationships. It's impossible to avoid sight altogether but try to maintain an embodied seeing, an inner visuality.
- When you start building the collage in relief or in three dimensions (like a dream catcher or a sculpted piece) ensure that you have prepared your temenos (see Chapter 3, Section B).
- Take your time and be in touch with your body as you work. You might need to linger with the scents, spend time with the textures and their memories, and listen to the music and recordings over and over. There's no rush.
- You'll know when you're finished, just as you knew when you were ready to begin.
- You may have something that is a compilation of senses that take you back and forward in time, but whatever the message, your aura will be embodied in the art piece.

A note on healing

Healing should have already begun through sensory collage making but there is always a need for consistent care of the self. The exercises below are an example of some ways that you can remain in touch with your body whilst emptying your mind and reducing dependence upon sight. The Zen Buddhists are particularly skilful at emptying the body and mind so that it blends with the universe in a oneness that is light and joyful. Zen monk Thích Nhất Hanh's many writings are immensely inspirational for an approach to 'non-self' (Nhất Hanh 1999).

Beyond sight: sound meditation

There are lovely sound meditation clips on YouTube or CDs that you can pur-chase but the essence of sound meditation for dreaming and healing is to keep it really simple. This sound meditation does not involve many instruments or sounds; there might only be one sound that guides you out of your mind.

Materials: One Tibetan singing bowl. Otherwise, there are already many sounds in the air and you don't need anything.

Process:

With a singing bowl:

- Ensure you are comfortable, wearing loose clothing, and barefoot is best.
- Select a soft mat that you can place on the floor to sit on. It's better to sit on the ground so that you are in touch with the earth. You may even prefer to sit outside in the garden under a tree on the grass.
- Sit in a position that allows your spine to be strong and straight with the rest of your body soft.
- If you have a Tibetan singing bowl, place it in front of you with its wooden mallet.
- Close your eyes and go into your breath, being aware of breathing in good-ness and breathing out all the unwanted stuff.
- Without opening your eyes, and maintaining a rhythmic breathing, reach out and strike the singing bowl firmly but gently on its rim with the mal-let, placing the mallet where you can reach it if you need it again, or keep it loosely in your lap.
- Focus on the sound of the bowl as it rings out, and resonates in your body.
- Notice and embrace the vibrations in your body. Larger singing bowls have stronger vibrations and deeper, more rooted tonalities, but the subtlety of smaller bowls with their higher pitch can be especially cleansing for the head. Smaller singing bowls can be placed on a small cushion (they often come with their own cushion) and held close to the head for head clearing. (If you hold a small singing bowl in your hand, the sound is absorbed into the hand and does not ring out.)
- Notice the sound as the chime fades very slowly becoming quite ethereal.
- Avoid striking the bowl again too soon, stay with the distant sound, the beauty of the path it left behind, and remember to breathe in and out, in an out – the out breath being most important as it cleanses you.
- Sometimes the drifting sound can evoke tears and feelings of sadness; if this occurs, just let the tears flow but stay in your breath which has its own calm-ing sounds and sensations.
- If there are any other sounds (and there usually are) in the room or the garden where you are sitting, *just notice them* and let them go; let them pass by with your breath.
- Don't open your eyes. If noise-sounds are persistent, strike the singing bowl again. Now let the singing bowl's sound be the one you focus on. In the

process the other sounds will lose their place in the hierarchy of sound. This will allow you to accept that all sounds are a part of this world but we don't need to focus on all of them, nor let them intrude upon our psyche.

- Follow the ring of the singing bowl in the same way as before, let it wash over and through you.
- Continue with this sound meditation as long as you need to; focussing on one sound should clear away all the noise in your head and leave you feeling light and joyful, whilst also remaining grounded with the earth.

Without a singing bowl:

- Try to ensure that all noisy appliances are turned off. Some can't be helped (like the refrigerator). Don't worry if you can't quieten absolutely everything, it is impossible; part of sound meditation is to rise above disturbance.
- Prepare yourself in the same way as above but now without the singing bowl.
- Close your eyes and be in and with your breath as above.
- Now notice all the sounds in the room, outside the room, in the garden and beyond the garden walls.
- If inside, there may the whirring of a ceiling fan or the sound of the refrigerator and outside it might be a water fountain, the sound of dry leaves rustling or green tree leaves brushing; there may also be bird calls and the hum of insects. There may be the patter of rain on a roof or dripping down windows, the sounds of wind whistling or even howling. There may be distant or close voices, the sounds of traffic or trains in the vicinity. All these and more are possible and they are part of our life.
- Whilst you sit with your breath becoming aware of the sounds that are sounds outside of your own head, the noise in your own mind will be drowned out by the external sounds which should bring relief.
- Select one sound if you feel it is comforting (sometimes the whirring of a fan inside or the dripping and bubbling of a water fountain outside work well as sound foci).
- The other sounds will still be there but they will disappear into the background and you may no longer even hear them. If they pop back into your sound sphere, just notice them *as sounds* and not for what they represent; do not name them because that engages cognition. This might be difficult at first but it's wonderful when you give yourself permission not to dwell on something. So for me the sound of a car revving is not something I can meditate on but, if it enters my sphere, I just notice it as sound, not as a car engine. This is liberating. But for another person the deep gurgle of an engine creates a pleasing resonance in the belly; sound-love is personal.
- Stay with your chosen sound whatever it is and let it wash over and through you without analysing it.
- Do this for as long as you need to.

Practices of silence and acceptance

This is also a valuable technique for bringing on sleep. Once you feel you have a good grasp of sound meditation, you can move onto silence. Practices of silence can take place anywhere and anytime that you feel is appropriate. Just as many people might cut down on sugar and fat in their diet, practices of silence can reduce unnecessary talking. Of course this allows you to listen more intently but sometimes you also need to regulate the amount of listening you can do.

Practices of silence are for you to find inner and outer peace. Silence is a necessary strength and is not just a negation of speech, it is a state of being and learning. This approach to silence is reminiscent of ancient mystic practices but also of some contemporary contemplative practices.

> Mystical silence is not simply a failure or a refusal to say anything, but it is instead a therapeutic strategy for approaching God. Thus, under certain conditions, silence might be the most appropriate response, because it is only in silence that any possible meaning can be found.
>
> (Zembylas 2004, p. 197)

Materials: Your own breath.

Process:

- Some places and situations bring silence upon us. These are usually vast and sublime like the desert, the ocean, some works of art, cathedrals and temples.
- If you are fortunate enough to be in one of these sublime places then incorporate your sound meditation techniques so that you are listening to the music of silence.
- The place will speak to you with its own sounds. Let it fill your body and feel your body resonate with the sound waves of silence.
- In usual day-to-day life, consider silence as your companion and select a time when you need to be quiet. It might not always be appropriate to close your eyes.

  - Be in your breath.
  - Follow the technique of sound meditation (without a singing bowl) above but avoid focussing on anything and let all the sounds 'just be sounds' so that they all wash over you and drift away.
  - There may be a persistent sound or voice that intrudes upon your silence, this noise could even be in your own head; breathe deeply, and when breathing out actually feel that sound blowing away.
  - To reach a true silence of the mind is not always easy, but acceptance is a more effective approach than resistance. Try greeting the voices or ideas in your mind, just with a smile as one would in passing someone on a walk but without stopping to engage in conversation.

○   Be very careful to stay in the rhythm of your breath. You are creating a beautiful void for your silent self which should become more calm, light and joyful with each exhalation.

Come out of your silence when you are ready and you'll find yourself feeling more kindly towards the world and instilled with more strength to cope. Additionally you should be more impervious to visual scrutiny from the external world.

Going for a walk and sense harvesting

The last time I went for a walk on a track in the Australian coastal shrub, I committed myself to a reduction of sight. I wanted to gather the sensory effects of my walk and retain those that were healing but discard those that were unpleasant. For example, I harvested the following senses: the joyful sound of children playing; the 'sheek, sheek, sheek' of the piping shrike (native Australian bird); the cool water splashed on my face at the water tap and its subsequent tickly evaporation on my skin; the difference between soft hot sand, massaging pebbles and spiky cool grass on the soles of my bare feet when I had removed my shoes; and the salty sea taste in the air.

Materials: comfortable clothes and shoes, protection against the weather.

Process:

- Do not take a phone, a camera or note paper.
- Let someone at home know where you're going and how long you'll be as a precaution.
- Go alone or with a companion who is committed to walking and sense harvesting but not as a talking companion.
- Choose a safe route you know well so you don't have to think, and choose one with no traffic roads to cross.
- Begin walking with your 'eyes wide closed'; by this I mean that you do not use your eyes to look or study things, they're just to keep you from tripping or colliding.
- Commit to using your ears, skin, nose and heart on this walk.
- If it's not illegal, you might pluck a piece of rosemary from a bush or pick up a pebble or shell for their scent and texture.
- Notice everything, pleasant and unpleasant; notice particularly what happens in and on your body when you hear, smell or feel something.
- When you get home, and have refreshed yourself, prepare to make some artwork on the sensory stimuli and responses during your walk.
- Set the temenos and either add to a collage you've started or make something different. You might want to compose a piece of music based on bird song or construct a sculptural piece for your garden that is for moving through and feeling, rather than observing.

- You might also want to return to your dream journal and find a walking dream or a nature-based dream and then you can blend your lived experience with your unconscious in the art piece you make.

Sensory dream gardening

This is an activity that can come out of the above walk; however, it can also be a dream garden that you may need to plant. Planting a seed or seedling can be a small ritual event for you.

Materials: seedlings, seeds, pot(s), cuttings, a garden bed, good soil, watering can, small trowel and garden fork. If at all possible avoid wearing gloves or footwear. Being in touch with the earth can be more than grounding; in-depth psychology grounding facilitates an 'opening' of the world beneath one (Hillman 1979, p. 200).

Process:

- Return to your childhood or a time/place where you remember particular plants with fondness.
- Acquire those plants as cuttings, seedlings or seeds and prepare a pot or garden bed by immersing yourself in the processes, textures and aromas. Be careful not to breathe in potting soil that has been sealed because this is very harmful to your health.
- Ensure that your plant will have sufficient light or shade.
- Dig the hole slowly focussing on the depth, colour and texture of the soil. Pour in the appropriate amount of water to make a luscious mud and plant your seed or seedling at the required depth.
- Most plants like company so try to create a little community of friends in your garden patch or container. All plants invite other living creatures to them, birds and insects become part of their community. They all connect symbolically to each other and to you. You may also want to create a small remembrance garden with relevant herbs and shrubs to lost ones. This can be extremely helpful in the absence of a gravestone or the ashes of your departed.
- Let the act of gardening, planting, caring and reaping (herbs/vegetables/flowers) be one of love for yourself with nature.

Preparing and sharing a meal/food

Some years ago I was living in my head too much and in a role at work that caused me to develop neck problems and severe headaches. One weekend in the kitchen whilst making a sandwich, I reminisced for the time when I was a young woman on a farm making my own breads and jams. The aroma of the rising yeast and sweet apricots came back through time as did the wonderful feeling of kneading and pounding the dough. I let my head go and began to be guided by my body. Returning to bread making was just the beginning; it was followed by many other creative activities across all of my senses. So at the end of this final chapter, it's good to go back to the symbolic ritual of making and breaking bread together. Below is my oat seed bread example. Regard this as a slow-cooking exercise.

Materials and ingredients: large bowl; measuring jug; kitchen scales; wooden spoon; bread-baking tin; greased paper; cling rap; instant dried yeast sachet; raw brown sugar; salt; butter; warm water; raw rolled oats; unbleached bread flour; sesame seeds; pumpkin seeds; sunflower seeds.

Process:

- A warm day is best, but if it's a cold day adjust the heating to warm the interior; alternately find a warm spot in your home.
- Be comfortable, ensure your work surface is not too high. It's best to stand when bread making as you need your whole body to push down on the dough.
- Lay all your ingredients and materials out.
- Weigh 1 pound (4 cups) of unbleached flour into your mixing bowl.
- Add 1 level teaspoon of salt.
- Add 2 generous teaspoons of raw sugar.
- Add a quarter pound (1 generous cup) of raw rolled oats (don't use instant or quick cooking oats).
- Add quarter pound (1 generous cup) of combined sesame, pumpkin and sunflower seeds.
- Mix well with your hands, taking in all the textures and their wholesome symbolism.
- Rub in 1 heaped tablespoon of cold butter with your hands breaking the butter into tiny bits so that the dried mixture combines thoroughly with the butter.
- Open a sealed sachet of instant dried yeast (equals two rounded teaspoons). I prefer the sealed sachets because they have not had contact with light or moisture. Pour this into your bread mixture and mix everything together. Notice the aroma of the yeast which is a living thing that is now an active agent in your mixture.
- Have a small jug of about 2 cups of tepid water (not too hot as this kills the yeast) and *slowly* pour some into the bread mixture mixing with a wooden spoon.
- You may not need all the water, this all depends on the moisture in the air. I sometimes only need 1¾ cups of warm water.
- Put your hands into the bread dough to mix the water into the dry ingredients very well; you'll know if it needs more water but it's better to have a moist dough than a dry dough.
- The dough will stick to your hands but rub it off and keep mixing; eventually the ingredients will blend into each other.

- When the dough forms a ball, take it out of the bowl with your hands and lay it on a flat surface that is clear for kneading. You can lightly flour the surface first but the more flour you have, the more water you might need to add.
- It's likely that the insides of your hands will still be sticky with dough; just rub it out onto the bread ball and begin kneading. The more you knead the less sticky it becomes but have a little extra flour there in case it really is too wet.
- Pull the dough over itself with two hands and then push the base/heel of your palm into the dough. Use your body as you push down; you should soon establish a rhythm. Alternate your hands to balance your body action.
- Breathe with the dough as you knead, and notice the power of your body.
- Sometimes the dough needs more water or a little more flour and sometimes it needs more kneading than others. The dough is ready when you push your thumb into it and it responds by slowly rising or springing back (Figures 6.3, 6.4, 6.5).
- It's important not to let the dough become dry so first rinse out your mixing bowl with warm water, then butter the inside, and finally put the dough inside the warm moist buttered bowl.
- Also butter a large piece of baking paper (enough to cover the top of the bowl well) and put the buttery side facing the inside so that when the dough rises up it does not stick.
- Cover with cling rap or a lightweight moistened kitchen towel.
- Place in a warm spot but out of the hot sun or cold drafts. Too much heat will turn the yeast sour and too little will prevent the dough from rising. Also remember that you don't want the rising to be too quick.
- The dough will be ready to take out for another kneading when it has doubled in size.

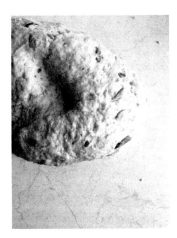

FIGURE 6.3 Kathleen Connellan (2018), *Springy Dough Ball.*

Author's own photograph.

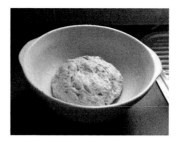

FIGURE 6.4 Kathleen Connellan (2018), *Dough in Bowl.*
Author's own photograph.

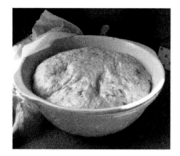

FIGURE 6.5 Kathleen Connellan (2018), *Dough after First Rising.*
Author's own photograph.

- When this is the case, put the dough back onto the kitchen table surface and knead it again until all the air bubbles are gone and the dough is light, springy and very responsive to your touch. The dough will seem smaller now and that's fine. Enjoy this dough that has its own life.
- Put it back into the freshly buttered bowl for a second rising. Place it in a similarly good position covered in the same way as before with buttered paper and cling rap or a towel to ensure it does not dry out.
- This second rising is usually quicker so when it has once again doubled in size, take it out.
- Once again knead all the bubbles out. Sometimes this just means a bit of punching and thumping which is good to relieve any residual frustrations that might be in your body. I usually have a bit of a chuckle when I do this. If you leave bubbles in your dough, the baked bread will have large holes and it will break when you try to slice it.
- At this stage the dough is beautifully springy.
- This time put the dough into a buttered bread loaf tin (Figure 6.6) and cover with buttered paper and a light towel or cling rap, placing it in a good warm-ish position on a table. This is the third rising.
- Turn oven onto hot, 200 degrees Celsius or 400 degrees Fahrenheit.

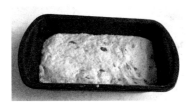

FIGURE 6.6 Kathleen Connellan (2018), *Dough in Loaf Tin after Second Rising.*
Author's own photograph.

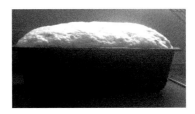

FIGURE 6.7 Kathleen Connellan (2018), *Dough in Loaf Tin after Third Rising.*
Author's own photograph.

- When the dough has risen to have a nice rounded top (Figure 6.7), not too high as too much will also cause the baked bread to break, and the oven has reached its temperature, take the paper and cover off the dough gently so it does not lose its shape and put it in the centre of the oven for about 20 minutes.
- Be mindful of the bread whilst it's baking; you don't want it to burn. You'll begin to smell the beautiful scent as it wafts through your home.
- After 20 minutes, peep in the oven to see if the top is golden brown. Sometimes it needs another 5–10 minutes; every oven is different.
- The bread is cooked when it's golden brown and if it sounds hollow when tapped. Take a moment to relish that satisfying resonant sound (see Plate 24 in the colour-plate section).
- Put the loaf onto a wire rack so that the bottom remains crisp and does not perspire.
- After a few minutes of cooling, it's probably ready to enjoy and share with gratitude.

Your own favourite

Materials: Your choice of ingredients, utensils and homeware or table adornment. Friends or family if you wish. Alternatively it may be that you just need a simple solitary experience and the practice of mindful eating.

Process:

- Go back to your childhood or a time/place where you remember a particular meal or food that was comforting and brought joy.

- Prepare your temenos. This is both in the kitchen and where the meal will take place. Aim for peace, calm lighting and harmony.
- Whatever foods you choose to prepare, ensure you are not rushed.
- Most good and fresh ingredients have distinct aromas and flavours, either alone or combined. Take your body and mind into a union with these and the feel of the ingredients in your hands as you work.
- Immerse yourself in the process and joy of creating a wholesome dish.

Solitary mindful eating or drinking

You can practise mindful eating or drinking in the same way as above with other foods/drinks. The entire process should be a ritual. After mindfully making and brewing your tea, you may want to encircle the warm mug with your hands, raising it to your lips to let the steam reach the pores of your face before your first slow swallow, which allows warmth to drift down into your body. Alternatively, with a beautifully coloured fresh peach, perhaps even plucked from your own tree, you can let its nature become a part of you. Hold it in your hands, enjoying its cool roundness and the astonishing blend of colours. Eating it outside beneath a blue sky, you can compare the colours of deep yellows, pinks and oranges. You can bite into the peach with gratitude and relish the wet sweetness as it covers your lips. A peach takes longer than a raisin (see below); it might even take half an hour to mindfully eat your peach, ending with its stone in your hand that is sometimes a rich brown. You may want to dry this superbly creviced stone and use it in an artwork.

Step by step with a single raisin or date

- Take a single raisin or date, you might need to pull it away from its sticky neighbours.
- Put it in the palm of your hand and sit down somewhere quiet and pleasant.
- Feel the light weight and presence of the raisin/date on your palm.
- Raise your palm to your nose and examine the fragrance in the fruit. This fragrance holds its life story.
- Now slowly open it with your hands to remove the stone or hard pips.
- Feel the stone or pips in your fingers and hands; notice the different texture between the hardness of the pip and fleshy stickiness of the fruit.
- Put the stone or seeds aside.
- Closing your eyes, put the raisin/date on your tongue slowly noticing it as it transfers its presence into the rest of your mouth's cavity.
- Turn it over with your tongue as it might stick to the roof of your mouth.
- Be mindful of it as it slowly disintegrates and dissolves with your saliva.
- Notice the spread of the abundant sweetness of this fruit.
- Swallow slowly, being aware of its pathway into the interior of your body carrying the natural sugars and minerals that are vital for your life.
- Open your eyes gradually and notice how eating slowly has a healing effect. Consider how this type of eating is like eating in a dream state.

Conclusion

This chapter has rejoiced in rekindling sensory memories. The natural world of growth and sentience includes humans in their most basic form. In this way the common phrase 'returning to nature' can mean letting go of the built and cultivated environment to be at one with our beginnings.

Sensory stimuli that take our bodies out of sight and into deep affect have immeasurable healing powers; struggles between controlled (hard) seeing and soft looking, need to be reconciled. Our eyes are too often linked to the exterior world of presumed scrutiny. Our heads are too often weighed down with the effects of presumed judgement. This chapter reminds us that our sensory body is larger and perhaps more capable than the cognitive mind. Our capacity to taste, smell, touch and hear gives us a sustained experience of the material and immaterial; simple things like truly listening to one beautiful or poignant sound and meditating on it, baking a loaf of bread and sharing its wholesome warmth with a friend, planting a seed and nurturing it to life. These are some of the things that the world of hard vision is missing.

Note

1 Some of the material in this chapter has been previously published. Excerpts are used, with permission, from the article 'Senses of memory in dementia care: the transcendent subject' published in *ATOL: Art Therapy OnLine* 9 (1) 2018, available at: http://journals.gold.ac.uk/index.php/atol/article/view/488/pdf

References

Bachelard, G. (1994), *The Poetics of Space: The classic look at how we experience intimate places*, trans. M Jolas, Beacon, Boston, MA.

Baird, A. and Samson, S. (2015), 'Music and dementia', *Progress in Brain Research*, vol. 217, pp. 207–235.

Benjamin, W. (1968), *Illuminations: essays and reflections*, trans. H Zohn, Schocken, New York.

Berger, J. (1972), *Ways of Seeing*, Penguin, London.

Bryson, N. (1988), 'The gaze in the expanded field', in H. Foster (ed.), *Vision and Visuality: Discussions in contemporary culture*, Bay Press, Seattle, WA, pp. 87–115.

Carruthers, M.J. (2007), 'The book of memory: a study in medieval culture', in M. Rossington Michael and A. Whitehead (eds), *Theories of Memory: A reader*, University of Western Australia Press, Perth, pp. 50–59.

Connellan, K. (2018), 'Senses of memory in dementia care: the transcendent subject', *Art Therapy OnLine*, vol. 9, no. 1.

Cox, B. (2015), *The Expanding Universe*, series 1, episode 2, television programme, ABC, 14 July.

Ede, S. (2013), 'Foreword', in F. Bacci and D. Melcher (eds), *Art and the Senses*, Oxford University Press, Oxford, pp. v – xvii.

Foster, H. (1988), *Vision and Visuality: Discussions in contemporary culture*, Bay Press, Seattle, WA.

Foster, H. (1995), *Compulsive Beauty*, MIT Press, Cambridge, MA.

Foucault, M. (1994), *The Birth of the Clinic: An archaeology of medical perception*, trans. A.M. Sheridan Smith, Vintage, New York.

Hillman, J. (1979), *The Dream and the Underworld*, Harper & Row, New York.

Johnson G.A. (2013), 'The art of touch in early modern Italy', in F. Bacci and D. Melcher (eds), *Art and the Senses*, Oxford University Press, Oxford, pp. 59–85.

Levine, S.Z. (2008), *Lacan Reframed*, Tauris, London.

Merleau-Ponty, M. (2002), *Phenomenology of Perception*, trans. C. Smith, Routledge, New York.

Nhất Hanh, T. (1999), *The Heart of Buddha's Teaching*, Rider, London.

Proust, M. (2006), *Remembrance of Things Past: Volume 1*, trans. C.K. Moncrieff, Wordsworth, London.

Rossetti, C. (1996), *Goblin Market*, Orion, London.

Sadie, S., with Latham, A. (eds) (1986), *Stanley Sadie's Music Guide: An introduction*, Prentice Hall, Englewood Cliffs, NJ.

Schama, S. (1995), *Landscape and Memory*, HarperCollins, London.

Stevens, C.J. (2015), 'Is memory for music special?', *Memory Studies*, vol. 8, no. 3, pp. 263–266.

Tomes, S. (2014), *Sleeping in Temples*, Boydell Press, London.

Tuan, Y.F. (1977), *Space and Place: The perspective of experience*, University of Minnesota Press, Minneapolis, MN.

Wade, N.J. (2013), 'The science and art of the sixth sense', in F. Bacci and D. Melcher (eds), *Art and the Senses*, Oxford University Press, Oxford, pp. 19–59.

Zembylas, M. (2004), 'The sound of silence in pedagogy', *Educational Theory*, vol. 54, no. 2, pp. 193–210.

CONCLUSION

The journey has only just begun. Now that you have a window in your wonder world of dreams and the tools to work with them, a rich creative future lies ahead. The aims of this book are to enter that dream world to search, discover, reflect, feel and then compose something healing. The process and the fruits of discovery are filled with paradoxes, which don't always need to be reconciled. This book has shown that the self in the wide world of consciousness is not alone. We are composed of differences which can be celebrated instead of negated. We have shadow and light selves, deep and surface selves, but this does not need to be a noisy complexity, it can also be a quiet simplicity. Ultimately it's the struggle of the soul and the taming of the mind. This requires silently being in the breath of the body and spirit. There are several exercises in this book that bring you back to your breath.

Practices that pay homage to distant pasts and eternal presence call for a care and knowledge of the self in the tradition of the Ancients. Give yourself permission to believe in a greater understanding that situates your self in a collective unconscious and spiritual communion within a vast universe. Reflections and exercises on being and longing take you to your dream place of rootedness which can simultaneously become the matter for making your enduring temenos. This will be a space of solace, a space to replenish a tired spirit and rejuvenate the body.

Your dreams may include movement. This psychic movement and the sensations of swimming in water, flying in air, climbing endless stairs or rugged mountains is shown to be part of an epic journey of searching and finding. It incorporates a flight of the soul from pre-birth to after life that reminds us of the fluctuations of existence. The dynamic aspect to dreaming and healing should bring energy, not fatigue. The exercises encourage you to recognise the paths of travel as well as the modes of moving. These are life's expeditions that may include the courage of escaping and leaving but also the endurance to return home with wisdom. Although only one chapter is exclusively devoted to movement, the whole book is about the circular rhythms of life's cycle. The will to live is emphasised; to be with Eros but to recognise Thanatos. There can be no life without death and no light without darkness; the blend is the mysterious miracle that feeds a creative spirit.

We live and dream in a world of things; the material world blends with the immaterial when we locate lost objects and hear their symbolic messages. Recognising loss and realising how the void may have been filled with objects or one specific object is crucial to healing the pain. Things are not always what they seem to be, and can be their absolute opposite. Even though there is again only one chapter devoted to the object in crisis and its ambiguities, the entire book deals with opposites. A simple household object can morph into something much more profound and take on the nature of a fetish. Transference from an object to the self or vice versa can help you rise above the pain of loss in a process of sublimation. This work can be done through the use of Dali's paranoiac critical method or the exquisite corpse method. Whichever tools are used to decipher dreamed and imagined objects or the symbolic identity of a tangible object, it's important to maintain a sense of humour. Allow yourself to smile at what looks ridiculous but nonetheless has something important to say. Even objects that assume fetish properties have light-hearted potential.

Just as joy and sadness contribute to dreamwork, so do all of our senses. The book takes a holistic approach to blending the mind and body, but it's easy to rely upon sight and neglect the remaining senses. Our eyes are usually closed when we're dreaming but even if they're open during daytime reverie, they are looking into a psychic space. The final chapter encourages us to turn our eyes inward and disregard the plethora of visual stimuli that crowd upon our daily lives; it also fosters a volume control of the noise inside the mind. Therefore with visual and auditory noises toned down, it is possible to use the senses as a source for healing. Taste, smell, touch and sound are each given prominence and elevated to bring wholeness to the self. There are many exercises that invite you to enjoy yourself and get right back into your organic body alongside, and within, the world of nature. Senses can be harvested to provide a rich trove for imaginative arts practice. Once the textures, tastes and harmonies of nature become ascendant, it's time to open your eyes again and you will notice the world differently. The quality of light and the warmth of the sun on water as you walk on the beach will join with the flutter of gulls' wings and the salty sweet smell of seaweed freshly washed up after a storm. You'll be able to see the sparkle of tiny shells and feel their grittiness beneath your feet.

This book is a balance between a scholarly and personally practical approach to dreamwork. I have combined art theory with psychology and philosophy. There is admittedly a leaning towards post-Jungian thinking which made sense as I progressed with the writing. We live in a spiritual and a social world; what we do and believe matters. James Hillman's (1992) claim that the world is getting worse despite a hundred years of psychotherapy is alarming. So too is Wolfgang Giegrich's (1991) implication that social systems now carry the shadow of civilisations. Therefore in the light of a real need to be connected with society, I hope this book is not seen as self-indulgent navel gazing, because our relationships with others are crucial for happiness. However we need to know and value ourselves before such relationships have enduring love. The theoretical sections devoted to poetry, art and profound reflection in the Symbolist and Romantic traditions also strive to bring postmodern relevance to a book that is geared towards deep knowing and real healing. Having said all of this, the theory is really a prelude to the core aspect of this book. This is essentially a book about making but one cannot make anything meaningful without the material resources and spiritual understanding.

A third of your life is spent in dreamtime; may it bring you hope and healing.

References

Giegerich, W. (1991), 'The advent of the guest: shadow integration and the rise of psychology', *Spring: A Journal of Archetype and Culture*, vol.51, pp. 86–106.

Hillman, J. and Ventura, M. (1992), *We've Had a Hundred Years of Psychotherapy and the World's Getting Worse*, HarperCollins, San Francisco.

INDEX

Entries in *italics* denote figures; entries in **bold** denote tables.

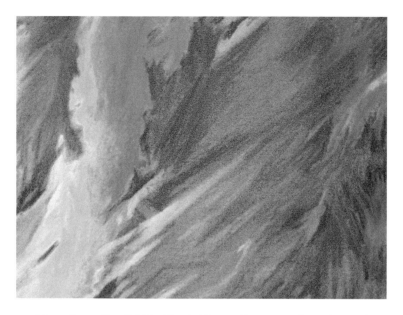

PLATE 1 Mary Connellan (2015), *Untitled Dream Version 1*, coloured pencil on card.
Reproduced with permission from the artist.

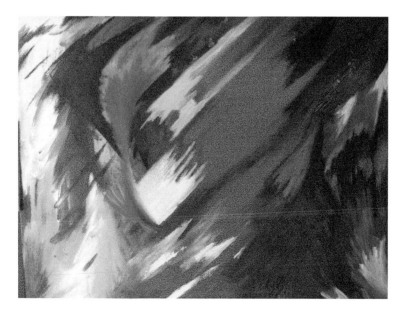

PLATE 2 Mary Connellan (2015), *Untitled Dream Version 2*, oil on canvas.
Reproduced with permission from the artist.

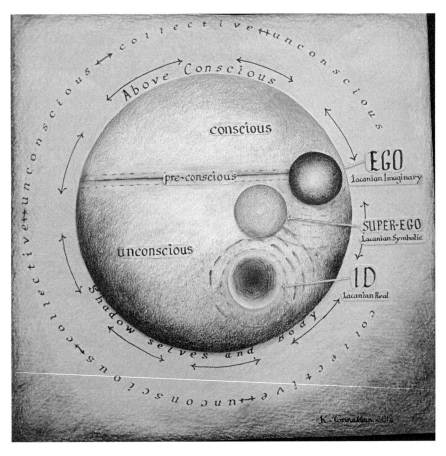

PLATE 3 Kathleen Connellan (2018), *The Self in Consciousness*, watercolour pencil, pen and ink on card.

Author's own artwork.

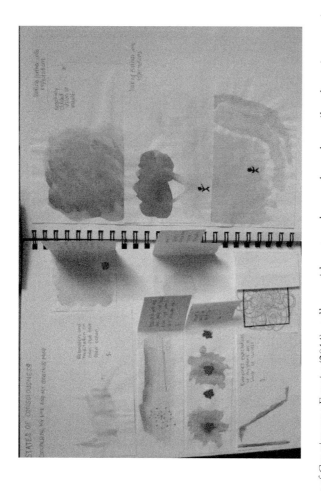

PLATE 4 Tandy's *States of Consciousness Exercise* (2014), collage with watercolour, coloured pencil and pen in an art journal. Reproduced in accordance with ethics protocols.

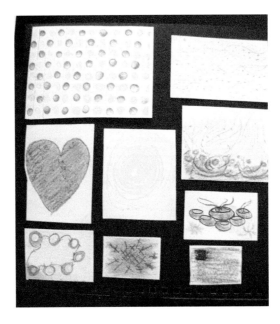

PLATE 5 Kathleen Connellan (2014), *States of Consciousness*, collage with watercolour, coloured pencil.

Author's own artwork.

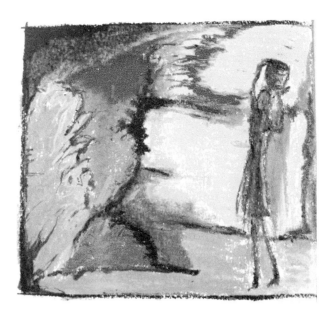

PLATE 6 Kathleen Connellan (2014), *Untitled Dream Image*, oil pastel on art journal paper.

Author's own artwork.

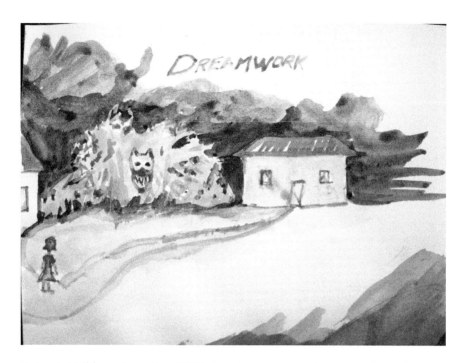

PLATE 7 Kathleen Connellan (2015), *First Dream*, watercolour on art journal paper.
Author's own artwork.

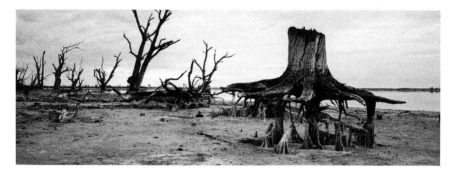

PLATE 8 Cumpston, Nici (2008), *Ringbarked II*, archival print on canvas, hand-coloured with pencil and watercolour.

Reproduced with permission from the artist.

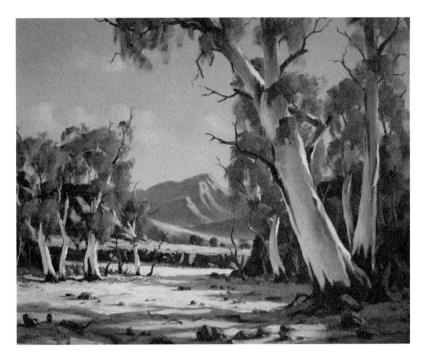

PLATE 9 Jansons, Ivars (1966), *Near Parachilna Gorge*, oil on board. Collection of the author.

Reproduced with permission from the artist's wife.

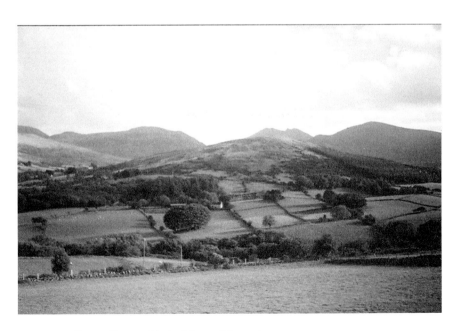

PLATE 10 *County Down with the Mourne Mountains.*

Photograph by the author.

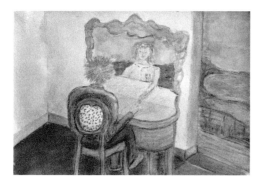

PLATE 11 *Joan's Mirror Dream* (2014), watercolour and coloured pencil on paper.

Reproduced in accordance with ethics protocols.

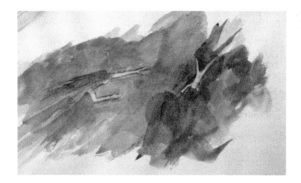

PLATE 12 Kathleen Connellan (2015), *Lost Child Swimming Dream*, watercolour on paper.

Author's own artwork.

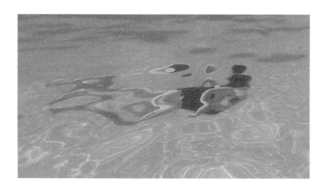

PLATE 13 Bridgette Minuzzo (2017), *Pool*, archival inkjet print. Still from slow-motion underwater video, Sanur, Bali. From the series 'Interesting places to swim'.

Reproduced with permission from the artist.

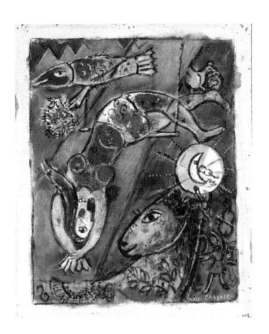

PLATE 14 Marc Chagall (1887–1985), *Blue Circus (Le Cirque Bleu)*, c. 1950, oil on canvas, image: 349 × 267 mm.

Presented by the artist to the Tate Gallery, London (N06136). Image supplied by the Tate London.

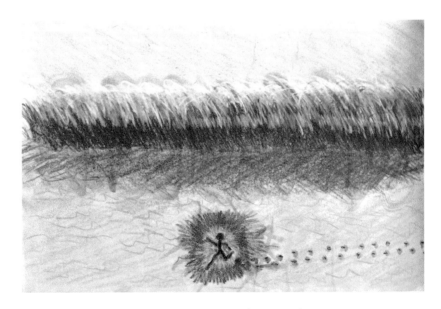

PLATE 15 *Joan's Dancing Dream* (2014), watercolour pencil on paper.

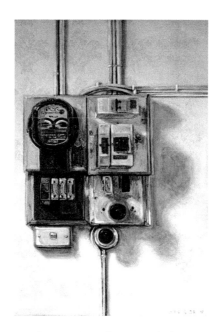

PLATE 16 Jasmine Symons (2018/19), *Stalker in a Balaclava*, oil on canvas, 52 × 78 cm. Reproduced with permission from the artist.

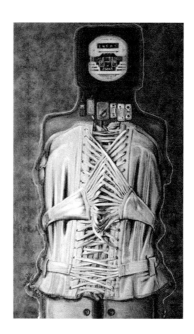

PLATE 17 Jasmine Symons (2012/13), *H-Armless (version 1)*, oil on linen, 66 × 112 cm. Reproduced with permission from the artist.

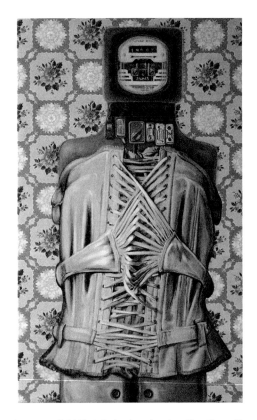

PLATE 18 Jasmine Symons (2013), *H-Armless (version 2)*, oil on linen, 66 × 112 cm. Reproduced with permission from the artist.

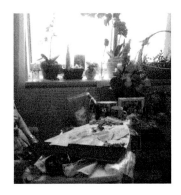

PLATE 19 Kathleen Connellan (2014), *Daisy's Collage Preparation*. Author's own photograph.

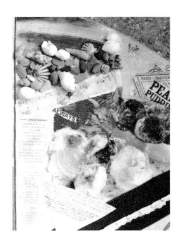

PLATE 20 Kathleen Connellan (2014), *Close-up of Daisy's Collage*.

Author's own photograph.

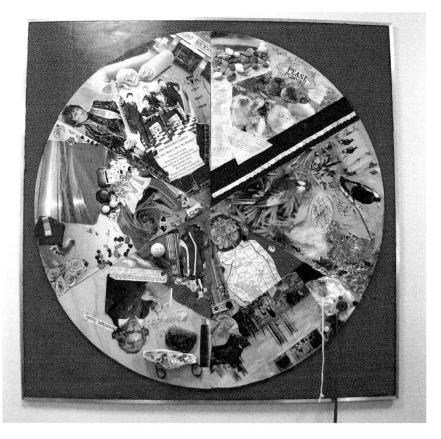

PLATE 21 Residents of an aged–care home (2014), *Combined Collage*.

Author's own photograph.

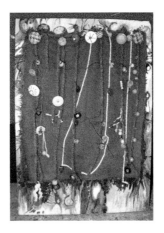

PLATE 22 Kathleen Connellan (2013), *Beads and Buttons*, textile and mixed media on board.

Author's own artwork.

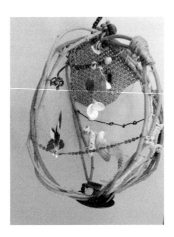

PLATE 23 Kathleen Connellan (2018), *Dream Catcher*, mixed media.

Author's own artwork.

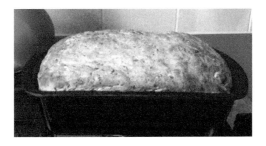

PLATE 24 Kathleen Connellan (2018), *Baked Loaf.*

Author's own photograph.